Disability Practice

Christine Bigby • Alan Hough
Editors

Disability Practice

Safeguarding Quality Service Delivery

palgrave
macmillan

Editors
Christine Bigby
Living with Disability Research Centre
La Trobe University
Melbourne, VIC, Australia

Alan Hough
Living with Disability Research Centre
La Trobe University
Melbourne, VIC, Australia

Purpose at Work
Franklin, ACT, Australia

ISBN 978-981-99-6142-9 ISBN 978-981-99-6143-6 (eBook)
https://doi.org/10.1007/978-981-99-6143-6

This Palgrave Macmillan imprint is published by the registered company Springer Nature Singapore Pte Ltd.
The registered company address is: 152 Beach Road, #21-01/04 Gateway East, Singapore 189721, Singapore

Paper in this product is recyclable.

This book is dedicated to people with disabilities, especially to those whose quality of life has been diminished, or who have been harmed, or who died as a result of service provision.

"To err is human, to cover-up is unforgiveable, and to fail to learn is inexcusable."
—Sir Liam Donaldson, champion of quality and safety

Foreword

The idea of modelling and measuring our quality of life might appear unnecessary to many people; a simple premise we enjoy unconsciously. In the same way that disability isn't immediately visible to everyone, despite around one in five Australians living with a disability. For many Australians their rights are invisible too because they enjoy unchallenged access to those rights, including the right to a high quality of life. The consequences of not upholding the rights of people with disability can be severe, as Christine Bigby points out in Chap. 2 of *Disability Practice: Safeguarding Quality Service Delivery* (*Disability Practice*). Instances of abuse, homelessness, unemployment and poverty are 'stark indicators of the failure to protect rights of people with disabilities' and highlight the significant impact of the systemic disadvantage they may experience.

One of the many issues *Disability Practice* articulates so well is the profound difference made to the lives of people with disabilities when their rights are respected and they are supported to exercise them through good practice and policy.

People are social creatures, biologically wired for cooperation, community and kinship. Social connections allow us to experience the full spectrum of feelings, from joy to love, grief and pain. They are also very motivating—more significantly than previously considered—and inform the value we gain from our lives.

If individuals naturally seek and prioritise social connections, does it not follow that inclusion and equity should be essential characteristics of a prosperous society? Looking at it another way, the social exclusion of some members of society disadvantages all of us.

These are some of the many questions *Disability Practice* raises for me. It is important such issues are discussed, particularly in the disability sector where we are increasingly guided by *quality of life* models and rights-based approaches to governance, policy design, support practice and service provision.

Disability Practice explores the many sentinels of the rights of people with disability and, perhaps most significantly, the quality of practice and the supports they receive. At the National Disability Insurance Scheme Quality and Safeguards Commission (NDIS Commission), quality is ingrained in our purpose of setting clear standards of expectation about the support provided to people with disabilities. High-quality support practice and service provision is a right and should be evident in every episode of service. Focusing on quality suggests that the design of services and delivery of all support should be guided by and aim to achieve the best possible outcomes, rather than guarding against the worst.

Disability Practice also explores the value of assessing disability supports and services against *quality of life* outcomes. Indeed, the quality of life model (Schalock et al., 2002) is an anchoring principle throughout this book as the eight domains identified in the model (see page 31) closely align to the UN Convention on the Rights of Persons with Disabilities (CRPD). Yet, the tools for measuring quality of life are much further advanced than those for measuring human rights. Again, this book clearly explains this approach and the virtues of using independence, freedom and inclusion—from quality of life models—as the guide to supporting people with disabilities.

The quiet power of this book is how it encourages a common-sense approach to supporting people with disabilities by essentially treating others as you would like to be treated. Don't we all appreciate feeling we matter, that we are included and our opinion counts? Don't we all want choice and control over how we live our lives, without having other peoples' values and preferences imposed on us? I contend, the answers to those questions are an instinctive and clear *yes.*

In the same vein, we must remember that the best disability services and supports will be designed *with* people with disabilities, not *for* them (see Chap. 12). After all, if you want to know what it's like to fly a plane, you ask a pilot. If you want to know what thoughts run through the mind of an athlete the moment they achieve Olympic or Paralympic glory, it's the athlete who'll articulate it best. The people who live the experience know how to achieve it, improve it or even avoid it. Listening to and finding ways to hear the preferences of people with disabilities with complex support needs is often the biggest challenge for supporters.

Disability Practice brings together some of the brightest minds in intellectual disability research, academia and advocacy. Their insights are not only deeply informed and critically reviewed, but they are also practical. Motivated by a shared desire to see people with disabilities supported to enjoy independence and active access to the communities of their choosing.

This book is a valuable resource for anyone supporting a person with disability in any capacity—as a family member or friend, policy maker, support worker or the executive manager of a service provider organisation. While it expertly offers an evidence-based exploration of the important issues regularly confronting people with disabilities and their carers, it also helps navigate a practical path through those challenges.

You will see that many of the chapters use case studies to reinforce the impact of issues being discussed, as well as objectively outlining the pros and cons of certain courses of action or inaction. Similarly, each chapter includes a useful summary of the main points discussed. In some instances, the ideas suggested could usefully be further explored in our own networks; I urge you to do this in your networks. I will be doing so in mine, particularly within our teams at the NDIS Commission, where we are committed to putting National Disability Insurance Scheme (NDIS) participants at the centre of all our decision-making.

In fact, one of the most encouraging features of *Disability Practice* is how it encourages curiosity as a way of building understanding. Each chapter and topic highlights the value of continued discussion and examination of how to support the rights and quality of life of people with disabilities, and offers practical guidance about how to support people based on their lived experiences.

Disability Practice deliberately focuses on adult Australians with intellectual disabilities, as this is the primary area of expertise for most of the book's contributors. As the largest single group of adult participants in the NDIS, most of whom have complex support needs, secondary impairments, and associated health or mental health conditions, all the research and recommendations referenced throughout *Disability Practice* are nonetheless instructive for the wider disability sector.

Complex issues are raised in this book and I suspect many, if not all of them, are well-travelled topics of conversation for those of us who are passionate about supporting people with disabilities. From understanding the social equity yet to be gained in health, lifestyle and economic and community participation, to ensuring the lived experiences of people with disabilities are automatically considered in the development of policy and support design. From building trusted relationships with transparency, engagement and people-centred practices to the creation of individualised support that ensures people with disabilities have the independence and choice they seek and deserve.

I am delighted to share that this book is available electronically as a free and accessible resource, with thanks to generous donations. *Disability Practice: Safeguarding Quality Service Delivery* is a thoughtful and intelligent resource designed to help us all. I encourage all family, friends, carers, disability service providers and their workers to take advantage of the knowledge and guidance offered freely in this book. Because, sometimes it's the most obvious questions that are the hardest to answer, but this book helps close the gap.

Tracy Mackey, NDIS Quality and Safeguards Commissioner
NDIS Quality and Safeguarding Commission
July 2023

Penrith, NSW, Australia — Tracy Mackey

Contents

Notes on Contributors

Sian Anderson, is a senior lecturer at the Living with Disability Research Centre, La Trobe University, Melbourne. Sian is the coordinator of disability practice courses at La Trobe University and has published on issues of community participation and inclusion, self-advocacy organisations, stigma and social identity.

Tal Araten-Bergman, is a senior researcher at the Living with Disability Research Centre, and senior lecturer at School of Allied Health, Human Services and Sports, La Trobe University, Melbourne. Tal has published on issues related to adults with disabilities' quality of life, disability policy and practice, service planning and family relationships across the life course.

Christine Bigby, is a professor and Director of the Living with Disability Research Centre, La Trobe University, Melbourne, and visiting professor at the Tizard Centre at the University of Kent. The focus of Chris's work is policy issues, programme effectiveness and frontline practice that supports quality of life outcomes for people with intellectual disability. She currently serves as President of the Australasian Society for Intellectual Disability.

Kathy Ellem, is a senior lecturer at School of Nursing, Midwifery and Social Work, the University of Queensland, Brisbane. Kathy's expertise includes participatory research with people with mild/borderline intellectual disability, with a focus on their interaction in the criminal legal system, self-advocacy for people with intellectual disability, and transition to adulthood. Kathy is keen to influence positive change in social work practice with this group.

Laura Hogan, is a General Manager Operations at the Centre for Disability Studies, and research affiliate in Sydney School of Health Sciences, University of Sydney, Sydney. Laura has extensive experience working with people with intellectual disabilities and complex support needs across the lifespan as an Occupational Therapist, supervisor, and manager. She is also a doctoral student at the Living with Disability Research Centre, La Trobe University, Melbourne.

Alan Hough, is an adjunct professor at the Living with Disability Research Centre, La Trobe University, Melbourne, and Director of Purpose at Work, Canberra. Alan has published on issues of disability service provider governance, quality and safeguarding, and regulation.

Lincoln Humphreys, is a lecturer at the Living with Disability Research Centre, La Trobe University, Melbourne. Lincoln has published research on organisational culture in group homes and developed training resources on Active Support and Practice Leadership.

Teresa Iacono, is Professor of Rural and Regional Allied Health at the Living with Disability Research Centre and Rural Health School, La Trobe University, Bendigo. Teresa is an academic and researcher, with publications in developmental disabilities across the lifespan, mainstream inclusion and complex communication needs.

Aaron J. Jackson, is a research fellow at the Living with Disability Research Centre, La Trobe University, Melbourne. Aaron has made significant contributions to disability studies by exploring fathering, care, and ethics within the realm of cognitive disabilities. His work not only challenges traditional gendered understandings of care and emotional labour but also provides valuable insights into the complex moral and ethical dimensions of life for those living with disabilities and their families.

Jade McEwen, was a research fellow at Australian Institute of Family Studies, Melbourne. Jade is a researcher, evaluator and policy analyst with expertise in measuring the congruence between intended outcomes and practice. Jade's previous work explored the way in which service quality is monitored in disability services and its adequacy as a mechanism for the prevention of violence and abuse.

Vivienne C. Riches, is a clinical professor, senior research fellow, psychologist at the Centre for Disability Studies, Affiliate at the University of Sydney, Faculty of Medicine and Health, Sydney. Fellow of the Australasian Society for Intellectual Disability (FASID), inaugural Lien Ling Chow Visiting Professor in Education, National Institute in Education, Nanyang Technological University, Singapore 2022–23. Interests include intellectual disability and employment, vocational training and transition, mental and emotional health and well-being and staff development.

Jane Tracy, is an Honorary Associate at the Living with Disability Research Centre, La Trobe University, Melbourne, and Murdoch Children's Research Institute, Melbourne. Jane is a medical practitioner who has worked for over 30 years to improve the healthcare provided to people with intellectual disabilities through a range of clinical, educational and research activities.

Jemma Venables, is a lecturer at the School of Nursing Midwifery and Social Work, the University of Queensland, Brisbane. Jemma uses qualitative methods to capture the experiences of marginalised children, young people, and their families as they engage with services to enhance policy and practice responses. Her work is particularly focused on young people's transitions from out-of-home care and the rights of children, young people and families engaged in child protection systems.

List of Figures

List of Tables

CHAPTER 1

Introduction

Christine Bigby and Alan Hough

This book is about turning visionary policies about the rights of people with disabilities into reality in their everyday lives. It is a guide to knowledge for designing quality services and to the practices needed to deliver enabling support to people with disabilities. The core argument of the book is that the quality of disability services and support rests on good practice—the moments of interaction between people with disabilities and services when knowledge is applied and principles become actions. Thus, we understand practice as conscious self-aware actions by support workers, managers or professionals where they apply knowledge, theories, principles and skills in real-life situations. Yet too often practice goes unnoticed and unmonitored, as paperwork—policies and procedures—dominates the attention of managers and expected practice remains abstract and ill defined.

C. Bigby (✉)
Living with Disability Research Centre, La Trobe University, Melbourne, VIC, Australia
e-mail: C.Bigby@latrobe.edu.au

A. Hough
Living with Disability Research Centre, La Trobe University, Melbourne, VIC, Australia

Purpose at Work, Franklin, ACT, Australia
e-mail: alan@purposeatwork.com.au

C. Bigby, A. Hough (eds.), *Disability Practice*,
https://doi.org/10.1007/978-981-99-6143-6_1

Policies and procedures are necessary to scaffold the delivery of services but are not sufficient for delivering quality support and safeguarding the rights of people with disability. Delivering services and support to people with disabilities cannot be proceduralised in the same way that it can be for making widgets. Standardised procedures ensure widgets are uniform, a consistent size and density—an indicator of quality. In contrast, delivering services and support requires 'standardised individualisation'—that is, systematic ways of working, as a team, in a programme, as a support worker, to understand and respond to each person's individual needs, preferences and potential risks to safety. This means the minutia of support looks different for every person reflecting their individuality—an indicator of quality. For example, in the context of accommodation services, standardised individualisation might mean; policies requiring a one-page profile capturing essential information about how a person communicates and the support they need to be engaged; procedures requiring every worker on every shift to be aware of this information; and training policies ensuring every worker has the skills to use that information in their practice—the way they interact with the person.

Good practice relies on the continuous judgements of workers and managers as they bring together and apply, in a unique combination, the values, skills, and knowledge necessary to meet the needs and preferences of each individual they support, at a specific time, in a specific context. This book is written for those charged with this task, from CEOs who create the conditions for good practice to direct support workers who carry it out. It will also be useful to professionals involved in advising disability services or delivering specialised support to people with disabilities, and to further and higher education students studying disability. This book is written to be accessible to non-academic readers.

Background

In Australia, the introduction of the National Disability Insurance Scheme generated unprecedented growth of disability support services and interest in the support necessary for people with disability to be fully included in society. Funding for services has doubled since 2013 as the Scheme has rolled out. Disability service is the fastest growing sector of the workforce, creating one in four new jobs. Growth is underpinned by the rights-based paradigm of the United Nations Convention on the Rights of Persons with Disabilities, which prioritises equal citizenship and inclusion of people with disability in all aspects of society.

The years of benign neglect of the disability sector have created major challenges to the sector's capacity to deliver quality services to support the policy intentions of the NDIS. Indeed, the Royal Commission on Violence, Abuse, Neglect and Exploitation of People with Disability systematically uncovered entrenched practices of abuse and neglect that undermine people's human rights. In the past work in disability has been low status. This together with the absence of a dominant profession leading practice has meant, until very recently, there has been scant research to inform the design of services and staff practice. Where research does exist, the transfer of knowledge from universities to providers has been a matter of chance.

Organisation of the Book

Written by leading practice researchers, this book fills a major gap by translating research and practice wisdom into the knowledge and practice needed to design services and to prepare staff to deliver enabling support. Most chapters focus on a distinct quality of life domain and consider:

- Why is this domain of quality of life important, and what disadvantages do people with disability face in this domain?
- What are the roles of support services in improving quality of life in this domain?
- What evidence is there about the design of services and the practices necessary to deliver quality support in this domain that disability service providers need to know?
- What do disability service providers need to know about other related service systems in order to maximise benefits in this domain for the people they support?

The book's primary focus is adults with intellectual disabilities. They are the largest single group of adult disability service users, many of whom have complex support needs, secondary impairments, and associated health or mental health problems. They are arguably among the most disadvantaged and neglected groups of people with disabilities, who require support across their life course in all life domains to exercise their human rights. Quality services are particularly difficult to achieve for this group. They are also the group for whom the voices of strong allies are needed alongside their own to ensure their individual and collective needs are represented to governments and service providers.

The context of this book is Australian, but much of the content around design and practice for quality services will be relevant to a wider international audience. The book is concerned with issues of quality and safeguarding in service provision. More general issues for people with disabilities, such as structural and economic disadvantage and intersectionality, or for organisations, such as management theories, are out of scope unless they are immediately relevant to a chapter's focus.

Ideally the book should be read as a whole, but each chapter is also written so it stands alone and can be read separately. For ease of reading, we have used minimal referencing and included a concise set of take-home messages at the end of each chapter.

Chapter 2. 'Thinking About Disability: Implications for Practice' by Christine Bigby introduces the diversity of people with disabilities and the merits of different models of disability for informing practice. She also reviews disability policy, individualised funding models, such as the NDIS, and the eight domains of quality of life.

Chapter 3. 'Building Strong Foundations: Listening to and Learning from People with Intellectual Disabilities and Their Families' by Aaron J Jackson and Christine Bigby explores the importance of the voices and perspectives of people with intellectual disabilities to service provision. The authors highlight what service providers can learn from actively listening to individuals with intellectual disabilities and emphasise the critical role of family in the lives of some service users, particularly those with severe or profound intellectual disabilities.

Chapter 4. 'Supporting Community Participation' by Christine Bigby, reviews different ways of supporting community participation. Through examples, she illustrates different programme designs, support worker skills and organisational features necessary to provide quality and individually tailored support for participation by people with intellectual disabilities.

Chapter 5. 'The Importance of Economic Participation for Quality of Life' by Vivienne Riches identifies the barriers and opportunities for people with intellectual disabilities to get and retain jobs of their choice. She describes the most effective employment models and good practices from across different employment programme types.

Chapter 6. 'Relationship-Based Practice with People with Mild Intellectual Disabilities Who Have Been Socially Marginalised and Excluded' by Kathy Ellem and Jemma Venables illustrates how disability support workers, organisations and service systems can support authentic and caring relationships with people with mild intellectual disabilities. They argue that relationship-based practice provides the context in which this group can build individual capacity, knowledge and resources to navigate the challenges of everyday life.

Chapter 7. 'Supporting Engagement in Everyday Life at Home and in the Community: Active Support' by Christine Bigby tackles the reasons for poor quality of supported accommodation services and presents evidence that when staff consistently use Active Support the people they support have higher levels of engagement and a better quality of life. She lays out the essential elements of Active Support and the frontline managerial practices, such as Frontline Practice Leadership, and organisational features necessary to embed it in services.

Chapter 8. 'Healthy Lifestyles and Primary Health Care' by Jane Tracy and Teresa Iacono reviews why people with intellectual disabilities often experience poor health. They then focus on the roles of disability services and support workers in both contributing to optimal health through direct support for individuals and supporting their interactions with health systems.

Chapter 9. 'Supporting People with Complex and Challenging Behaviour' by Laura Hogan and Christine Bigby uses case examples to illustrate how to apply evidence-informed principles to support people with complex needs. They propose a framework for the practices that must be in place to ensure the quality of life of adults with intellectual disabilities and challenging behaviours in the context of accommodation supports.

Chapter 10. 'Support Planning with People with Disabilities' by Tal Araten-Bergman explores the purposes of support planning, from determining funding and setting broad life goals to creating detailed blueprints for delivering a specific type of support. She sets out the principles, thoughtful processes and person-centred actions necessary to avoid support planning being a meaningless paper exercise.

Chapter 11. 'The Right to Participate in Decision Making: Supported Decision Making in Practice' by Christine Bigby reviews the contested nature of substituted and supported decision making and proposes a principled approach that puts the person's will and preferences at the centre of all decisions. She alerts service providers to the varied landscapes of decision making and explains an evidence-based practice framework for supporting decision making that is applicable across all types of decisions and contexts.

Chapter 12. ' 'Nothing about us without us.' Including Lived Experiences of People with Intellectual Disabilities in Policy and Service Design' by Sian Anderson and Christine Bigby reviews different approaches to tapping into the expertise of people with disabilities from their lived experiences of disability and the practices that are most effective for working together with people with intellectual disabilities. They consider some of the unresolved issues that support workers, managers and policy makers grapple with to further the rights of people and ensure there is 'nothing about us without us'.

Chapter 13. 'Organisational Culture in Disability Accommodation Services' by Lincoln Humphreys explains the significance of culture in disability services and its influence on staff behaviour. The chapter explores the characteristics of culture in good and poor quality services and considers actions that organisations and frontline managers may take to change and maintain culture.

Chapter 14. 'Building Quality and Safeguarding into Disability Service Provision' by Alan Hough and Jade McEwen demystifies what workers and service providers should do to deliver high-quality and safe supports while acknowledging the complexity involved. They argue that strategies should be integrated into standard ways of working rather than approached as a box-ticking exercise disconnected from day-to-day practice.

We acknowledge the generous donors who enabled us to make the book open access. We also thank the authors of each chapter for their commitment to this project. We hope that in some small way this book contributes to improving the quality of life of people with disabilities as readers use the evidence and practice wisdom it captures to improve the design of disability services and quality of support they provide.

CHAPTER 2

Thinking About Disability: Implications for Practice

Christine Bigby

People with disabilities are a very diverse group, which is reported to make up around 15% of the world's population. The group includes people with functional limitations, impairments or health conditions which differ in terms of cause, severity and impact on their everyday lives. It includes people with different diagnostic labels, personal characteristics and identities, who live in different social and economic contexts. Despite these differences, people with disabilities share common experiences of disadvantage many of which are created by society and compromise their quality of life and exercise of rights.

We think about disability in different ways—how it is described, measured and understood. This can be confusing when we talk about how many people have disabilities. More importantly perhaps, different ways of thinking about disability lead to competing views about the types of laws, policies, services and practices that should be put in place. For example, whether to talk about people with disability in general or specific impairment groups, what language to use ('disabled person' or 'person with a

C. Bigby (✉)
Living with Disability Research Centre, La Trobe University,
Melbourne, VIC, Australia
e-mail: C.Bigby@latrobe.edu.au

C. Bigby, A. Hough (eds.), *Disability Practice*,
https://doi.org/10.1007/978-981-99-6143-6_2

disability') and whether government disability policies should be directed at segregation, social inclusion, care or supporting the exercise of human rights. All of these are subtly different.

This chapter explores some important conceptual issues. The chapter reviews differing descriptions and socio-demographics of disability. It compares and contrasts some of the ways of thinking about disability and describes the context of disability practice. The chapter points to the value of *Both/And* thinking for practice (that is, holding multiple perspectives about disability at the same time) and the potential dangers of *As If* thinking (accepting as true something that is known to be untrue to further social change) (Appiah, 2017; Smith et al., 2016). The author's expertise is in research with people with intellectual disabilities: where examples are given, they will usually relate to intellectual disability. The circumstances of people with intellectual disabilities are sometimes different to those of people with physical and sensory disabilities and can provide an important way of testing ideas about disability services, programmes and practice.

Describing Disability

Governments use broad descriptions of disability from international bodies, such as the World Health Organisation (WHO) or the United Nations (UN) to show who is included in the disability group. The WHO description of disability is part of the International Classification of Functioning (ICF) and can be summarised as:

> Disability is a difficulty in functioning at the body, person or societal level, in one or more life domains, as experienced by an individual with a health condition in interaction with contextual factors. (Leonardi et al., 2006, cited in Bickenbach, 2019)

The UN Convention of Rights of Persons with Disabilities (CRPD) describes disability as an evolving concept and Article 1 states that:

> Persons with disabilities include those who have long term physical, mental, intellectual or sensory impairments which in interaction with various barriers may hinder their full and effective participation in society on an equal basis with others. (United Nations, 2006, Article 1)

Very simply both the WHO and CRPD describe disability as the interaction between individual characteristics and social contexts. However, the language, purpose and values of each of these descriptions are different. The ICF uses the language of health. Its purpose is a universal classification system, a model for understanding the creation of disability and ways of improving human functioning. In contrast, the CRPD's description of disability does not use the language of health. It uses the language of humanity and equity rather than functioning. The values in its description are explicit and its purpose is not scientific understanding but advocacy and pointing to the social change needed to achieve equality and human rights for people with disability.

Counting Disability

Leaving models of disability aside for the moment, governments and service providers need more precise definitions of disability to collect information about people with disabilities, develop laws or design social programmes. Creating precise criteria and pinning down exactly the number of people with disabilities is not straightforward—it requires decisions about who is included. For example, governments may want to use broad criteria when they report national expenditure on disability to the UN or plan at the population level for health, education or transport services. Governments may want to use narrower criteria to determine individual eligibility for programmes such as transport subsidies, income support or social care. For example, the commonly reported figures that 18% of the Australian population or 4.4 million people have disabilities of whom 32% (1.4 million) have severe or profound disabilities are very different from the much smaller figures of 610,502 people eligible participants in the National Disability Insurance Scheme (NDIS, 2023) or 746,000 recipients of disability support pension (AIHW, 2022).

Knowing who has been included is important when figures about disability are reported, as they may refer to:

- a nation's whole population and the prevalence data (the number or proportion of the population with disabilities),
- particular age groups and the age-specific prevalence data (proportion of a specific age group with disabilities) or

- data about specific subgroups of people with disabilities, categorised, for example, by type or severity of disability, location or eligibility for or use of particular types of services.

How the data to calculate figures about disability were collected and by whom are also important. In Australia, for example, the Survey of Disability Aging and Carers (SDAC) conducted by the Australian Bureau of Statistics (ABS) is the gold standard for identifying and capturing information about disability (AIHW, 2022). It provides comprehensive and detailed data about people with disabilities of all ages across the whole of Australia. The survey sample is large and representative. The survey uses 120 questions to identify disability. They reflect a functional definition: 'having at least one limitation, restriction or impairment to everyday activities which has lasted for at least 6 months'. The survey specifies ten types of limitations such as self-care, communication, property maintenance and meal preparation. When people surveyed are identified as having disabilities they are categorised by severity (mild, moderate, severe or profound) according to how many and what types of activities they need help with. They are also grouped into six disability groups (sensory and speech, intellectual, physical, psychosocial, head injury and stroke and other).

Many of the other surveys that give data about people with disabilities focus on subgroups in terms of age (children or youth), location (state or locality) or service sector (housing, health, education). Criteria used to identify people with disabilities often rely on self-identification, and differ from those of the SDAC, particularly in terms of the number of limitations a person has and length of time they have had them (see AIHW, 2022).

Age is a critical dimension for counting how many people have disabilities. The prevalence of disability increases exponentially by age. On some counts 50% of people with disabilities are aged 65 years or older, and people 85 years and older are twice as likely to have disabilities compared to those aged 65–69. Sometimes reports separate people by age; labelling those under 65 years as people with disabilities and those over 65 years as older people. At other times reports put all age groups together and use the label people with disabilities. If only people below the cut-off for 'older' are included, the number of people with disabilities is much smaller 9% rather than 18% of the Australian population or 2.2 m rather than 4.4 m. As this illustrates, administrative decisions can change who and how many people have disabilities. Interestingly, in Australia service systems are divided on the basis of age and the aged care and disability sectors have different standards and funding.

Disadvantage and Disability

People with disabilities do much worse on all indicators of disadvantage compared to people without disabilities. This is the case no matter how the group is defined or the data collected. Table 2.1 compares adults with and without disabilities and, where the information is available, people with severe or profound disabilities, on key indicators of disadvantage. The source of these data is Australian Institute of Health and Welfare (AIHW, 2022) which explains in detail the criteria used and how they were collected. All figures have been rounded up or down.

These data show that people with more severe levels of disabilities experience even greater disadvantage. More detailed data show that people with psychosocial or intellectual disabilities often experience more disadvantage than other groups of people with disabilities. For example, people with intellectual disabilities aged under 65 years are less likely to use most health services, other than dental, than all other disability groups and have much higher rates of unemployment (AIHW, 2022).

Large-scale government surveys that collect representative or statistically robust samples are important for planning and gaining broad snapshots of people with disabilities compared to other groups. Such surveys do not include hard-to-reach groups—such as those with severe cognitive disabilities—or provide in-depth pictures of people's lives. This is what scholarly research does, often using smaller and more targeted samples of subgroups of people with disabilities. Some researchers use qualitative methods, asking people to talk about their experiences or observing them, which gives a richer picture of what life is like for people with disabilities. For example, focusing just on death rates of people with intellectual disabilities, researchers showed the much shorter life expectancy of this group and the high rate of deaths that could have been avoided by proper health care compared to the general population (Heslop et al., 2014). All types of data are valuable and provide different insights into the group of people with disabilities.

There are dangers of concentrating on disability status alone. Focusing only on disability hides what is referred to as *intersectionality*. That is the other personal characteristics or identities people with disabilities have that may compound the disadvantages they experience as a person with disability. For example, data shows the higher rates or different types of disadvantages experienced by people with disabilities who are women, from

Table 2.1 Comparing adults with and without disabilities on key social indicators

Social indicator	*Adults with disability 25–64 years*	*Adults with severe or profound disability*	*Adults without disability*
Health			
Self-rated fair or poor health	42%	62%	7%
Insufficient physical exercise	65%		48%
Delay in access to GP	8.7%		4.1%
Delay in access to dental care	32%		20%
Material wellbeing			
Government payment primary source of income	43%	69%	7.9%
Low income	20%		9%
Financial stress	38%	51%	27%
Cannot raise $3000 within one week in an emergency	42%	28%	10%
Went without meals in a week	8%		2%
Education#			
Studying post-school	9%	2%	15%
Barriers to post-school study or work goals	64%		48%
Intending to go to university	48%		66%
Economic participation			
In the labour force	53%	27%	84%
Employed	48%	24%	80%
Unemployed	10%	13%	5%
Part-time work	41%	52%	32%
Satisfied with job	54%		61%
Discrimination and safety			
Not satisfied with personal safety	12%	22%	5%
Lifetime experience of sexual violence*	21%		10%
Social connections			
Experiences social isolation	17%	24%	9%
Experiences loneliness	28%	37%	16%
Member of a club	28%	20%	36%
Dissatisfied with local community	39%	46%	27%
Difficulty getting places	23%		17%
Living situation			
Lives alone	19%		8.%
Not satisfied with home	14%	20%	8%
Moved for health reasons	8%		1%
Life satisfaction			
Satisfied or totally satisfied	51%		69%

* Centre of Research Excellence in Disability and Health (2021)

includes young people 16–25 as well

culturally and linguistically diverse backgrounds, First Nations people, live in remote and rural locations, or identify as LGBTQI (AIHW, 2022).

The following sections move away from describing disability and counting how many people have a disability. These sections consider different models or ways of understanding disability. Each has its own way of understanding why people with disabilities experience the disadvantages already described and how to tackle these disadvantages.

Value of Understanding Different Models of Disability

Models are ways of making sense of complex things and help to organise our thinking. Understanding models of disability is not just an intellectual exercise. Each model emphasises different aspects of disability, giving different perspectives about what might be important to people with disability, what needs to change to support them and different types of policy and practice. Understanding different models of disability is helpful because each model provides insights and suggests strategies that are not mutually exclusive and can be used together. The three models considered are the social model of disability, the individual deficit model of disability and the emerging critical realist model.

These models are described in the following sections as *ideal types* to show the differences between them; in practice the types are not always as distinct from each other.

Social Model of Disability

Definition

The social model of disability was developed in the late 1970s by UK disability activists. Many were people with physical disabilities with first-hand experiences of individual deficit models of disability (discussed in the following section). The social model separates impairment from disability, defining impairment as “lacking part of or all of a limb or having a defective, limb, organ or mechanism of the body” (Oliver & Barnes, 2012, p. 22). In contrast, disability is conceptualised as:

> The disadvantage or restriction of activity caused by contemporary social organisation which takes little or no account of people who have physical impairments and thus excludes them from participation in mainstream of social activities. (Oliver & Barnes, 2012, p. 22)

In this model disability is created by the way society is organised, as it is not designed to include people with impairments and excludes them. For example, disability results from the design of infrastructure such as buildings and public transport, the organisation of the labour market, the design of services such as education and health, and stigmatising social attitudes that devalue and exclude people with impairments. Hence people with impairments are disabled by society and use of the term disabled people is appropriate. This model has a strong human rights approach.

What Needs to Change

Concentrating solely on disability rather than impairment, the social model shows that changes are needed to the way societies operate rather than changing people with impairments. Social model thinking focuses attention on extrinsic rather than intrinsic factors: that is, it looks outwards to society rather than inwards to people with impairments. It provides strong and clear but very broad messages about what needs to change to include people with impairments in society.

Disability activists using the social model initially emphasised change to improve physical and sensory accessibility and social attitudes. For example, removing obstacles such as the lack of alternatives to stairs to enter buildings, public toilets that were too small for wheelchairs or lack of audible signals at road crossing. Much later, advocates applied social model thinking to people with intellectual disabilities and ideas of cognitive accessibility. For example, the obstacles to access posed by complex digital systems to answer phone calls that require responses to many automated options before reaching a customer service person, electronic touch on touch-off cards for transport systems or complex text as the primary form of communication by service systems.

One of the guiding questions in applying social model thinking is how does the problem facing a person with impairment stem from their social situation and how can this be changed?

Questions Important to Applying the Social Model of Disability
Is the reason a person cannot use public transport because they use a wheelchair for mobility or because of the design of buses and trains?

Is the reason a person does not use a local gym because of their lack of social skills and motivation to keep fit or is it because of the way other patrons stare at them, the unwelcoming attitudes of the receptionist and the need to produce a driving licence to prove their identity?

Is the reason a person cannot secure a well-paid job because of their lack of skills and poor literacy or because the labour market system values jobs requiring complex skills and multi-tasking more highly than those requiring little training or repetitive tasks?

Some of the changes suggested by social model thinking are increasingly taken for granted in Western societies. These include, for example, provision of lifts, ramps, access to all facilities for guide dogs, requirements for physically accessible public buildings and facilities, anti-discrimination laws and multiple methods of communicating in public broadcasts. They are indicative of the success of using the social model to advocate for change, although some would argue such changes only begin to scratch the surface of what needs to change.

Pros and Cons

The social model promotes leadership by people with disabilities in policy and service provision, recognising that people with disability are experts about their own experiences. Universal human rights are integral to the model. The social model helps to identify the common interests of people with disability by focusing attention away from different types of impairments. This avoids splitting people with disabilities into different interest groups, bringing them together as one group to advocate for change. The clear messages of the social model are easily adapted to single-issue advocacy. On the other hand, the broad-brush nature of the social model does not give detailed prescriptions about the many and different types of change needed to make society accessible. It is also criticised for neglecting changes that are more specific to people with intellectual disabilities.

It is further criticised for paying too little attention to impairment. Particularly, neglecting what is often seen as the intrinsic and direct impact of some impairments such as pain, restricted movement or capacity for learning or quick thinking. Making a distinction between impairment and focussing on disability means that impairments are seen as medical issues, and associated with individual genetics, lifestyle or accidents rather than the organisation of society. Consequently, social model thinking gives little attention to the social conditions that may create impairments, such as poverty, pollution or unequal access to health care.

At its most pure, the social model envisages a society that is inclusive of all people, where everyone can participate regardless of their impairments and where separate provisions are unnecessary for people with impairments. The extent of change required to achieve this would be so far-reaching that inclusion as a concept would no longer be meaningful—all people would be included all the time (Clapton, 2009).

Implications for Services

The primary focus of the social model is changing all levels of society, including the organisation and delivery of services. It focuses policy on making mainstream services accessible but also the provision of individualised personal care and support to enable people with disabilities to participate. The model has a strong rights perspective, and advocates for public funding of services to assist people with disabilities to have greater independence, choice and control over their lives, and to be treated with respect. The early social model activists founded the 'Movement for Independent Living' that promoted the right to personal assistants, to assist people with disabilities to achieve independence and dignity. They envisaged that personal assistants would be directed by people with disabilities as would the organisations that employed and managed this workforce. This movement foreshadowed individualised funding for services as a way of promoting choice and control of personal care and support by people with disabilities.

The social model holds key messages about people with disabilities leading and directing both services and service organisations. It makes assumptions that people with disabilities can self-direct support and consequently devalues training and skills needed for the practice of direct support work. However, at the practice level, if applied well the social model does draw attention to ways of working that support physical and cognitive accessibility. For example, supporting decision-making by making information accessible or supporting participation in meetings by slowing the pace and taking breaks.

Individual Deficit Model of Disability

Definition

Individual deficit models of disability (referred to as individual models) are often used to show differences to the social model of disability. There is no one body of writing associated with individual models. They focus on individuals and the impact of impairments on a person's health and functioning (physical, cognitive or psychological). The connection between impairment and disability is direct and straightforward—impairment leads to disability—therefore people are disabled by impairments rather than society. These models emphasise 'defective limbs, organs or mechanisms of the body' (Oliver & Barnes, 2012, p. 22). It is argued that it is these 'defects' that restrict or limit an individual's ability to perform activities or participate in society. Advocates refer to this as a deficit approach, as it highlights what individuals with impairments cannot do and how they are different from 'normal' people. Disability is seen as a tragedy within individual deficit models. In the past application of individual models led to the separation of people with disabilities from society and segregation (putting them together in one place) so they could be educated, treated or protected, or in some instances so society could be protected from them.

What Needs to Change

Use of individual models sometimes still leads to specialist or separate services. But more recently, these models are also used to find ways to improve the functioning of individuals with impairments. For example, optimising physical movement, improving skills, sight, hearing or speech or assisting a person to adjust psychologically to the experiences of acquiring an impairment or practically to impairment-related restrictions. This may involve medical treatments, allied health therapies, training and education or supply of prostheses (artificial limbs), hearing aids or glasses. It may also mean using knowledge about a person's health or genetic condition to improve their health, ensure they get appropriate and timely treatment, avoid future risks of poor health or understand behaviour. The models can, for example, help us in understanding that, among other things, Prader-Willi syndrome is associated with an insatiable appetite that means that no matter how much a person eats they will not feel full, or that Down Syndrome is associated with high risk of premature ageing and early onset of Alzheimer's dementia.

The primary focus of change to improve quality of life is the individual, but may also extend to change in their immediate environment. This may involve modifying a person's home to take account of impairments and make it safer, by installing rails or ramps or providing equipment or technologies to make tasks easier to do, such as smart devices that raise or lower blinds, provide sound reminders about medication or give spoken instructions for operating machines. These types of change are tailored to each individual and referred to as adjustments or accommodations. They are not necessarily concerned with system-wide changes to accommodate all those with similar needs. The type of change foreshadowed in individual models relies heavily on the expertise of allied health, medical and psychological professions.

Pros and Cons

Application of individual models may have a direct and positive impact on a person's wellbeing and quality of life and assist their participation in activities and social interactions. The focus is on reducing or removing the direct negative effects of impairment—reducing pain, mental anguish or improving mobility. By attending to impairments, a person's health or functioning may be improved, and actions may be taken to respond to identified health risks, treatments or explanations for behaviour that improve quality of life. For example, increasing the skills of a person with intellectual disability may increase their chances of getting a job (in tandem perhaps with social model approaches of reducing discriminatory attitudes), and understanding genetic factors associated with Down syndrome may sensitise those around a person to their higher risks of heart defects to prompt regular monitoring and early interventions.

On the other hand, individual model thinking draws attention away from what people with disabilities have in common and the disadvantages this group experience. The focus on individual differences may create competition for scarce resources, such as specialised services, research or therapy. Individual models are also criticised for medicalising disability, devaluing or stigmatising people with disabilities, by marking them out as special and different. The emphasis on specialist needs, treatment, knowledge and adjustments has at times led to provision of poorer quality services compared to those available to the rest of the population. For some people this model is associated with a readiness approach, that is, delaying participation until a person has the necessary skills or physical capacity to participate rather than providing immediate assistance to participate that compensates for difficulties in functioning, such as individual support or equipment.

Implications for Services

Individual models do not have a strong rights perspective, but they are concerned with ensuring all people have opportunities to function to the fullest and participate in society. The focus of policy and services is on improving functioning. This means investment in research to find evidence about the best types of interventions. This might be medical treatments or therapies, technologies to replace tasks and support functioning, or methods of teaching skills. Policy will be directed to development of specialist services for specific diagnostic or functional groups and the training and credentialing of professional groups to deliver services.

At the practice level expert knowledge about the needs of different groups of people with disabilities and nature of impairments is emphasised. The focus is on working with individuals and using professional skills to provide individualised care and support and adjust immediate living or working contexts.

Critical Realist Model of Disability

Definition

A critical realist model of disability is evolving. It is a realist model because it accepts the reality that, for example, some people have bodies that hurt or brains that function differently to others. It is a critical model because, like the social model, it challenges the idea that disability is a deficit. The model has a strong rights-based values stance, hence, the name 'critical realist model'.

A critical realist model is characterised by interactions between factors intrinsic and extrinsic to individuals. In this model disability is understood as the:

> Interaction between individual and contextual factors which includes impairment, personality, individual attitudes, environment, policy, and culture. ... [Disability is created through] the combination of a certain set of physical or mental attributes in a particular physical environment within a specified social relationship, played out within a broader cultural and political context which combines to create the experience of disability for any individual or group of individuals. (Shakespeare, 2014, pp. 77–78)

It considers a much wider range of factors about individuals and society than the social model. The critical realist model is sometimes also described as an interactional or relational model, particularly in the Scandinavian literature. It is sometimes confused with bio-psycho-social or social-ecological models which also look at individuals and social contexts but do not have such a strong rights stance.

What Needs to Change

Concern with the interaction between impairment and social structures as well as other individual and contextual factors make this model more complex than either social or individual models. It has multiple targets for change. It draws attention not only to individual or collective experiences of people with disabilities but also to the issues common to particular subgroups such as the difficulties with decision-making often shared by people with cognitive impairments but not experienced by people with physical or sensory disabilities. This highlights that people with different types of impairment often face different obstacles and helps to identify the different strategies needed to remove them.

Examples of the Application of the Critical Realist Model of Disability

Most societies use written words and visual signs as the main way of sharing information. This relies on visibility—people being able to see words and signs. It creates an obstacle for people with vision impairment who cannot see words or signs.

The strategies to remove this obstacle are both structural and individual. They include using additional ways of conveying information. Such as spoken words, sounds or tactile symbols. For example, sounds at traffic lights, braille on automatic teller machines, and technology for individuals to turn digitally written words into spoken form, such as JAWS (software that reads information on screens aloud). These types of strategies are now common in some societies.

A critical realist model highlights that strategies such as these will not be effective for all people with impairments. Some people, with different kinds of impairment or identities, face more complex obstacles created by reliance on written words. For example, translating words into spoken language will not be effective for people with vision impairment who are also deaf. Neither will direct translation from written to spoken words be effective for some people with intellectual disabilities. For this group the obstacle is not visibility of written words but keeping up with the speed that people talk and understanding the meaning of what they say. Some people with intellectual disabilities need a different type of translation, one that slows the pace and simplifies the language be it spoken or written.

Even translation to makes things more understandable will not make information accessible for those with profound intellectual disabilities. For this group it is the very use of symbols and abstract concepts that pose the obstacle to access. For this group strategies for making information accessible have to be individualised, relying on skilled workers or others who know a person well to judge the relevance of the information to the person's situation or interpret their preferences about options it contains.

Pros and Cons

The critical realist model avoids the type of *either/or* thinking of the social and individual models that concentrate either on society or impairment. It uses *both/and* thinking, paying attention to both impairment and society. The model suggests that it is "only by taking different levels, mechanisms and contexts into account" that the complexity of disability can be understood and action taken (Danermark & Gellerstedt, 2004, p. 350). Going back to the example above, strategies to remove obstacles for a person with intellectual disability and low literacy created by reliance on written words may include training to improve the person's literacy *and* regulations that require translation of all written information into plain English.

The critical realist model is concerned with *what exists* and the ways *we think about it*. The model does not try to hide the intrinsic disadvantages of some impairments. For example, some disadvantages are real and intrinsic to intellectual impairment including difficulties with time or abstract concepts, problem-solving, making decisions or assessing risk. Some of these disadvantages will not be removed by changing either the individual or their social context. This would require fundamental changes to society. They may however be reduced by providing good support or changing social contexts. Critical realists argue what is important is how we (our society) think about people with intellectual impairment. They argue that people with intellectual impairment should be valued, regarded as equal human beings with the same rights to dignity and respect as all others in society. What we think (social values) influences government actions and the distribution of resources. For example, government investment in learning and development programmes, individualised support and changing social systems to be more inclusive may not completely remove the disadvantage of intellectual impairment but will strongly influence people's quality of life. Thus, the disadvantage experienced by people with intellectual impairment stems from, among other things, the interaction of impairment with social values. Too often in the past the intrinsic disadvantages of intellectual impairment have been made worse by social values that dehumanise and devalue people with intellectual disabilities. They have been considered as 'not rational', and experienced being stigmatised, feared, excluded or discriminated against. These experiences are not intrinsic to intellectual impairment they are created by interactions between impairment and society and can be removed by changing society's values.

Implications for Services

The implications of the critical realist model for practice and service design are far-reaching. It points to the importance of considering all possibilities to reduce disadvantage experienced by people with disabilities. It helps to understand that different goals, types of interventions and strategies lend themselves to different levels of society including the individual directly. The critical realist model shows what might be achieved at which level of society and assists in identifying all possible strategies when making judgements about the best use of resources and where to intervene.

For example, it helps to make judgements about when it is appropriate to explicitly acknowledge the differences between people with disabilities and when to concentrate on what the group has in common. At the risk of using jargon, the concepts of ***differentiation*** and ***dedifferentiation*** are useful here. Differentiation distinguishes between people with disability on the basis of the type of their impairment. Dedifferentiation on the other hand says that no distinctions should be made. Judgements about which strategy is appropriate must take account of the context and level of potential intervention. The NDIS provides a good example.

Differentiation and Dedifferentiation in the NDIS

The campaign for the NDIS aimed to bring significant change to disability policy and disability service systems. The target for change was at the national level. It used a dedifferentiated approach that glossed over differences between people with disability. This approach successfully unified people with disability by highlighting what they had in common.

A dedifferentiated strategy was much less successful at the level of practice in the NDIS, for things such as planning with people for individualised packages of support. Here a differentiated strategy would have worked better. To plan effectively for supports to enable people to exercise their rights to choice and control in their lives, planners needed to understand the differences between people with disabilities in terms of communication, decision-making, and support needs and know about impairments. Planners lack of knowledge led to poor quality plans and frustration on the part of people with disability. For example, people with genetic conditions were reported to feel disrespected by staff who asked inappropriate questions about how long their condition would last.

Critical realist and social model thinking share similarly strong perspectives about the rights of all people with disability regardless of the severity or nature of their impairment. Critical realists take an approach to practice that emphasises people's strengths. But they also consider it is important to understand the *real* impact of a person's impairments to make sure they get the right type and amount of support they need to exercise their rights. Thus, assessment and planning with people with disabilities and people that know them well is considered, and drawing on multiple sources of information including expert knowledge is important to getting the right support (see Chap. 11). Critical realists avoid using *as if* ways of talking that represents people with disability *as if* they do not have impairments or *as if* their impairments are less severe than they are. This type of misrepresentation is often used to demonstrate everyone is equally human and may help in advocating for rights and status. But at the practice level it gets in the way of understanding support needs and the types of adjustments a person may require to participate successfully.

Similarly, critical realists are more likely to promote *interdependence* rather than simply independence: that is, how people rely on each other and the importance of relationships to the quality of care and support. They also recognise the long-term and continuous support needs of some people. This helps to avoid representing people's support needs *as if* they are short term or transitory. This often happens in behavioural support services, where, for example, good support and trusting relationships may help to reduce a person's incidents of challenging behaviour, but this does not mean the person no longer needs a high level of support. Too often if support is reduced it is likely that challenging behaviour will return.

At the practice level critical realist thinking is more likely to argue that recognising individual or group differences is important so that support is tailored to every individual or the group they belong to. This type of thinking brings together many of the strategies offered by individual and social models, but by emphasising *both/and* thinking encourages judgement about the strategies that are most appropriate for each person or each group at a particular time in a particular context. At the policy level critical realist thinking is more likely to emphasise issues common for all people with disabilities to secure the redistribution of resources and high-level change to ways of doing things that are necessary to achieve equality of human rights for people with disabilities.

Table 2.2 summarises three models of disability showing the perceived advantages, shortcomings and implications for policy and practice of each model.

Table 2.2 Summary of disability models

Disability definition	*Perceived advantages*	*Perceived shortcomings*	*Implications for policy and practice*
Social model Disability is the "restriction or disadvantage caused by contemporary social organisation that takes little or no account of people with impairments and excludes them from participation in mainstream activities" (Oliver & Barnes, 2012, p 22).	• Attention to changing social structures and processes that create disadvantage. • Simple and strong messages for advocacy. • Promoting common interests and solidarity among people with disability and diverting attention from individual differences. • Leadership by people with disabilities. • Human rights perspective. • Individual support for personal care or participation needs controlled and directed by people with disabilities. • Focussed on independence, choice, control and dignity of people with disability.	• Focuses more on physical and sensory accessibility with less attention to cognitive accessibility and types of obstacles experienced by people with intellectual disabilities. • Neglect of the downsides of some impairments such as pain or fatigue. • Broad and simple messages about change rather than detailed prescriptions for change at multiple levels. • Blind to other intersecting identities of people with disabilities. • Unrealistic expectations that society can be organised for universal access given competing types of obstacles and change people with impairments require. • Blind to issues of interdependence and supports some people need to exercise choice and control.	**Policy** • National and State laws and regulation about discrimination, accessibility, such as design of buildings, public places, public transport, mainstream services. • Systemic change to social processes to accommodate people with disability, such as mandated training for professions across all service systems including legal, health and financial systems as well as social care. • Building systemic approaches into programmes to taking account of needs of people with disability, such as flexibility for longer consultations. • Mechanisms to fund individualised care and support as a right. **Practice** • Adjustments to ways of working, such as slowing down, taking breaks, producing and using multiple modes of communication, ways of interactions. • Personal assistants directed by people with disabilities.

(*continued*)

Table 2.2 (continued)

Disability definition	*Perceived advantages*	*Perceived shortcomings*	*Implications for policy and practice*
Individual deficit model Disability is what accompanies impairment: the "physical or psychological concomitants of impairment" (Priestley, 1998, p. 75), and is portrayed as negative, marked by some sort of inferiority or loss for the individual.	• Identifying differences in individual needs. • Attending to direct and negative impact of some types of impairment. • Reducing health risks. • Improving individual functioning, skills or health. • Adjustments to environment based on individual need. • Specialisation and use of evidence and expertise.	• Focus on deficits. • Readiness approach: rehabilitation or learning enables the person to be ready in the future rather than supporting participation here and now. • Special and different provisions are often of poor quality or lead to exclusion or segregation. • Little attention to systemic change of the social structures and processes. • Dominance of professional and scientific expertise.	**Policy** • Focus on ways to improve functioning. • Investment in evidence-based interventions, such as medical treatments and therapies. • Investment in technologies to replace tasks and support functioning. • Investment in learning and teaching. • Investment in specialist services for specific diagnostic or functional groups. **Practice** • Importance of expert knowledge about needs of different groups of people with disability and nature of impairments. • Focus of professional skills for individualised care and support and adjustment of immediate social context.

Critical realist model Disability is the outcome of "interaction between individual and contextual factors which includes impairment, personality, individual attitudes, environment, policy, and culture" (Shakespeare, 2014, p. 77).	• Unpacks nuanced and complex nature of disability. • Promotes Both/And thinking able to incorporate aspects from social and individual models. • Recognises diversity within the disability group and similarities within subgroups. • Recognises that types of obstacles and thus changes needed depend on the types of impairment and other individual and contextual factors. • Attention to both impairments related and socially created obstacles and disadvantage. • Avoids *as if* thinking such as representing all people with intellectual disability as if they only have mild impairments which obscures different types of support needs. • Rights perspective.	• Facilitates complex understanding of disability. • Multiple potential strategies for change meaning there are no simple messages for change. • Requires judgements to determine appropriate levels of intervention and strategies. • Focus on deficits as well as strengths. • Requires skilled support to enable choice and control for some people rather than relying on only worker values or direction by people with disabilities.	**Policy** • Attention to potential for intervention and change at multiple levels—law, regulation, community and individual. • Multiple concurrent programmes and strategies for intervention focussed on system change to benefit all people with disability, for particular subgroups, and for individuals. • Mechanisms for individualised funding for care and support that include provisions to enable people with cognitive disability to use these effectively to exercise rights. • Investment in skills training for disability support workers, and practice leadership. **Practice** • Tailored to individuals based on knowledge about multiple facets of an individual and their social circumstances. • Emphasis on understanding of impairment differences and intersectionality. • Focus on interdependence and support relationships as well as independence and instrumental support.

Supporting Rights and Quality of Life

The overarching aims of disability policy and practice are to reduce the disadvantages experienced by people with disabilities: ensuring people have a good quality of life, can exercise their human rights and are protected from discrimination or abuse. Rights and quality of life are key indicators of success. They are broad umbrella terms which include other policy visions for people with disabilities, such as social inclusion, community participation, choice and control, independence and self-determination.

Rights

Rights have become more important since the United Nations adopted the CRPD in 2006. The CRPD is an international convention that aims to "promote, protect and ensure the full and equal enjoyment of all human rights and fundamental freedoms by all persons with disabilities, and to promote respect for their inherent dignity" (United Nations, 2006, Article 1). The CRPD sets out and explains the meaning of the human rights of people with disability in articles: statements that outline the purpose, definitions and principles of the convention. These include:

- Equality before the law without discrimination (Article 5)
- Right to life, liberty and security of the person (Articles 10 and 14)
- Equal recognition before the law and legal capacity (self-determination) (Article 12)
- Freedom from torture (Article 15)
- Freedom from exploitation, violence and abuse (Article 16)
- Right to respect physical and mental integrity (Article 17)
- Freedom of movement and nationality (Article 18)
- Right to live in the community (Article 19)
- Freedom of expression and opinion (Article 21)
- Respect for privacy (Article 22)
- Respect for home and the family (Article 23)
- Right to education (Article 24)
- Right to health (Article 25)
- Right to work (Article 27)
- Right to adequate standard of living (Article 28)

- Participation in political and public life (Article 29)
- Participation in cultural life, recreation, leisure and sport (Article 30)

Governments around the world that have signed up to the CRPD promote and protect rights through the types of strategies discussed earlier in this chapter that flow from various models of disability. They include for example:

- anti-discrimination and equal opportunity laws,
- policies requiring local governments and public bodies to make disability action plans,
- regulations about building accessibility,
- standards or guidelines for web accessibility or plain language,
- programmes such as supported decision-making and
- services and individualised supports to people with disabilities.

Abuse, homelessness, unemployment and poverty are stark indicators of failures to protect rights of people with disabilities. Positive indicators of rights are more difficult to find. Legislation and policy often assert people with disability have rights but this is rarely enough. Many people need resources and skilled support from family, friends or services to exercise their rights effectively. This is often referred to as putting policy into practice or making rights real. The outcome of a person exercising their rights also depends on individual preferences. For example, one person may use their rights to self-determination and to live in the community to choose to live with their parents into middle age, another may choose to live in a group home, and another in their own in a flat.

Quality of Life

In a similar way to Rights, *Quality of Life* provides a common language for talking about visions for life, and outcomes that might be expected from service systems. Although relevant to all people, the application and measurement of quality of life has been most comprehensively developed in the field of intellectual disabilities where international consensus about its eight domains has been reached (Schalock et al., 2002). Quality of life has eight domains that apply to everyone and everyone's quality of life looks different. The eight domains are:

- Interpersonal relations,
- Emotional wellbeing,
- Personal development,
- Physical wellbeing,
- Self-determination,
- Social inclusion,
- Rights,
- Material wellbeing.

While there is close alignment between quality of life domains and CPRD rights, tools for assessing or measuring quality of life are much further advanced. This means that for individuals quality of life may be a more useful indicator of success of legislation, policy or practices. Quality of life can be judged in various ways: against a person's own goals, against indicators tailored to the particular subgroup a person belongs to or, for some domains, against objective indicators. For example, using a method called goal attainment scaling, progress on each of a person's goals can be measured every six months, and scores compared over time (Shankar et al., 2020). Of course, this depends on how well goals were developed and reflect a person's preferences. However, this is a much more useful indicator of change than simply asking a person how satisfied they are with their life or their services, as most people are satisfied most of the time no matter what is happening to them (Schalock et al., 2002).

Table 2.3 further describes the eight domains and some of the indicators developed for people with more severe intellectual disabilities (Bigby et al., 2014). You will see that many of these rely on practice: that is, the quality of support a person receives.

Quality of life is an umbrella term that includes the aims of inclusion or choice that are often singled out in policy or mission statements of disability support organisations. Every service that delivers good support contributes to a person's overall quality of life but some services focus more strongly on some domains than others. For example, a community access service is likely to pay particular attention to supporting social inclusion and interpersonal relationships, compared to an advocacy service that will concentrate on rights and self-determination.

Table 2.3 Quality of life domains and exemplar indicators

Domain	*Indicators*
Interpersonal relations	**Individuals** • experience positive and respectful interactions. • are supported to have regular positive contact with their family. • know people other than paid staff and family.
Emotional wellbeing	**Individuals** • appear content with their environment, activities and staff support. • appear happy and take part relatively willingly in a range of activities with the right support. • are at ease with staff presence and support.
Personal development	**Individuals** are supported to • engage in meaningful activities and social interactions in various areas of their life. • try new things, experience success and develop their skills. • be competent and develop confidence and self-esteem.
Physical wellbeing	**Individuals** are supported to • have a good diet and regular exercise. • have access to regular health checks appropriate to age. • have pain or illnesses recognised and responded to.
Self-determination	**Individuals** are supported • to express preferences and make choices about their lives. • by someone who knows them well and can help others to understand their preferences. • to understand information through appropriate communication.
Social inclusion	**Individuals** are supported to • use local community facilities. • take part in activities with people with and without disabilities. • have a valued role, to be known or accepted in their communities.
Rights	**Individuals** • are treated with dignity and respect in all interactions. • have someone who advocates for their needs and interests. • have access to transport and community facilities.
Material wellbeing	**Individuals** • have their own possessions around their home. • are supported to manage their finances. • have access to sufficient funds to make purchases of their choosing.

Disability Services and Practice

Disability practice is the application of knowledge, values and skills to supporting people with disabilities to have a good quality of life and safeguarding their rights. Disability practice takes place in the context of services and programmes. For example, a support worker may be directly employed by a service user to assist them to participate in sport, they may work in a programme delivered by an organisation that provides leisure and recreation services for people with disabilities, or in a mainstream leisure service that is adjusting its programmes to include people with disabilities. A support coordinator or case manager may practice as a sole private practitioner, or as part of a support coordination service, or in a support coordination programme in a disability support organisation that delivers other programmes (such as supported accommodation or community access), or as part of a mainstream service such as the social work department of a public hospital. Together, services such as these make up health and community service systems. These systems are complex and shaped by government priorities, policy and funding. Some professional practices, such as social work, rely on a deep knowledge of service systems but most do not. Nevertheless, some understanding of the broader context of practice is helpful in seeing how the services a person receives fit together.

Health and community service systems have changed significantly in recent years. They are becoming more *person centred*, putting service users at the centre of everything they do and giving them greater control. In some parts of service systems the shift towards person-centeredness has changed funding arrangements from block funding of services to individualised funding. That is, rather than money going directly to organisations which decide what services to provide and who will use them, the money goes directly to individuals to spend on the services they choose. Individualised funding needs four elements:

- *Sufficient individual funding* for each individual to purchase the services they want.
- *Flourishing markets* where there are sufficient services available, which are of the type people want, in the places people want them,

so people can choose which services to purchase and change services if they are not happy with what they get.

- *Savvy consumers* where people with disabilities know what services they want, where and how to get them and are confident to manage and coordinate them and change services if they are not happy with them.
- *Effective regulators* that set and monitor the standards of services—preferably in an evidence-based or evidence-informed way—and promote compliance both by positive strategies to promote learning and improvement and by enforcement action when needed.

Of course, individualised service systems are much more complicated than this, and there are many other processes in each element. For example, individual planning is needed to determine the allocation of funding to each individual and once allocated to plan what to purchase; markets need to be encouraged to develop particular types of services or supply them in isolated places where demand is low; many people with disabilities need supported decision-making or advocacy to be good consumers and to articulate their needs, or choose and manage their services; and regulators must identify what information to collect about the quality of services, determine where to set standards and how to judge quality.

Most of these processes rely on skilled disability practice by those who work directly with people with disabilities and others who are important to them, who lead and supervise direct workers, and who design and manage programmes. The Australian NDIS is one of the most fully developed individualised funding schemes for disability services. It is administered by the National Disability Insurance Authority (NDIA) and almost all government funding for disability services is allocated as part of the scheme to individuals with disabilities to spend on the services they choose. This means that services rely on the NDIS money that each individual service user brings with them for all of their income. If they do not attract enough services users to cover their costs they will go out of business. There is now excellent material on the NDIA website that explains how the scheme works and a recent book by Cowden and McCullagh (2021) provides both description and commentary about the NDIS.

There are aspects of the health and community services system that are not suited to individualised funding. The individual consumers of some services are not easily identified and may be a wider collective of individuals, or be groups or communities. Thus advocacy, community development or projects to make mainstream services more accessible should continue to be funded directly by governments. It is also argued that governments need to play a significant role in strategic planning and commissioning of services, to ensure all the needs of people with disabilities are well understood and met rather than leaving this to markets alone. The NDIS is unique in this respect in that unlike some individualised schemes it directly commissions only a very few services although it does try to influence the market through price and policy.

Around the world health and community service systems are continually adjusting to meet the competing demands of economic sustainability, ideology and government priorities. There is no doubt that service systems influence the context and nature of disability practice but fundamentally the quality of practice and thus support for people with disabilities to have a good life relies on the knowledge, values and skills of those who carry out practice.

Take Home Messages

- People with disabilities are a diverse group who are significantly disadvantaged on all social indicators.
- The different ways of describing and measuring disability determines the size of this population which if you use prevalence is as large as 18% (4.4 m) of the population in Australia, or as small as 610,502 people who are eligible for the NDIS.
- Three of the most common ways of understanding disability are the social model, the individual deficit model and critical realist model—each gives different insights into ways of improving the lives of people with disabilities. Both/And thinking suggests that all of these are useful in disability practice.
- The social model emphasises the need for change to the structures and processes of society so be inclusive of people with disabilities, the individual model emphasises the finding ways to improve the functioning of individuals often through specialist services, and the critical realist model is concerned with the interaction between people with disabilities and society, focusing both on maximising individual functioning and development and adjusting the social structures of society to be more inclusive.
- The concepts of quality of life and rights are useful ways of thinking about what disability policy, services and practice are trying to achieve for people with disabilities.

References

AIHW. (2022). *People with disability in Australia 2022.* Australian Government.

Appiah, A. (2017). *As if: Idealization and ideals.* Harvard University Press.

Bickenbach, J. E. (2019). The ICF and its relationship to disability studies. In J. E. Bickenbach (Ed.), *Routledge handbook of disability studies* (pp. 55–71). Routledge.

Bigby, C., Knox, M., Beadle-Brown, J., & Bould, E. (2014). Identifying good group homes: Qualitative indicators using a quality of life framework. *Intellectual and Developmental Disabilities, 52*(5), 348–366.

Centre of Research Excellence in Disability and Health. (2021). *Nature and extent of violence, abuse, neglect and exploitation against people with disability in Australia.* A. Royal Commission into Violence, Neglect and Exploitation of People with Disability.

Clapton, J. (2009). *A transformatory ethic of inclusion: Rupturing concepts of disability and inclusion.* Sense Publishers.

Cowden, M., & McCullagh, C. (2021). *The National Disability Insurance Scheme: An Australian public policy experiment.* Palgrave Macmillan.

Danermark, B., & Gellerstedt, L. C. (2004). Social justice: Redistribution and recognition—a non-reductionist perspective on disability. *Disability and Society, 19*(4), 339–353. https://doi.org/10.1080/09687590410001689458

Heslop, P., Blair, P. S., Fleming, P., Hoghton, M., Marriott, A., & Russ, L. (2014). The confidential inquiry into premature deaths of people with intellectual disabilities in the UK: A population-based study. *The Lancet, 383*(9920), 889–895.

NDIS (2023). NDIS Quarterly Report to disability ministers.

Oliver, M., & Barnes, C. (2012). *The new politics of disablement* (2nd. ed.). Palgrave Macmillan.

Priestley, M. (1998). Constructions and creations: Idealism, materialism and disability theory. *Disability and Society, 13*(1), 75–94. https://doi.org/10.1080/09687599826920

Schalock, R. L., Brown, I., Brown, R., Cummins, R. A., Felce, D., Matikka, L., Keith, K. D., & Parmenter, T. (2002). Conceptualization, measurement, and application of quality of life for persons with intellectual disabilities: Report of an international panel of experts. *Mental Retardation, 40*(6), 457–470.

Shakespeare, T. (2014). *Disability rights and wrongs revisited* (2nd ed.). Routledge Publisher.

Shankar, S., Marshall, S. K., & Zumbo, B. D. (2020). A systematic review of validation practices for the goal attainment scaling measure. *Journal of Psychoeducational Assessment, 38*(2), 236–255.

Smith, W. K., Lewis, M. W., & Tushman, M. L. (2016). "Both/and" leadership. *Harvard Business Review, 94*(5), 62–70.

United Nations. (2006). *Convention on the Rights of Persons with Disabilities (CRPD).* UN General Assembly.

CHAPTER 3

Building Strong Foundations: Listening to and Learning from People with Intellectual Disabilities and Their Families

Aaron J. Jackson and Christine Bigby

Since the 1970s, the disability movement, led by people with disabilities, has played a key role in changing disability policy and service systems. People with intellectual disabilities have contributed to these changes but have not maintained a high profile. Too often they are not well supported to participate or are represented by families and other allies. The same is true of research and developments in disability practice and safeguarding, where perspectives of people with intellectual disabilities are underrepresented.

The new rights based policy approaches discussed in this book emphasise hearing directly from people with lived experience of disability about their experiences as service users to inform what policies need to change and how services should be designed. More funding is becoming available

A. J. Jackson • C. Bigby (✉)
Living with Disability Research Centre, La Trobe University, Melbourne, VIC, Australia
e-mail: Aaron.Jackson@latrobe.edu.au; C.Bigby@latrobe.edu.au

C. Bigby, A. Hough (eds.), *Disability Practice*,
https://doi.org/10.1007/978-981-99-6143-6_3

to scaffold support for people to speak for themselves and knowledge is growing about effective ways of doing this. These new directions are not intended to devalue the role of families and allies in representing their perspectives about what is important to people with intellectual disabilities. Rather these trends aim to distinguish, more clearly than in the past, the views of people themselves from those committed to their wellbeing.

Leadership and presence of people with intellectual disabilities in Disabled Person's Organisations and public campaigns is increasing, and raising their profile as one of the largest group of adults who use disability services. For example, in June 2022 the leadership and contribution of three people with intellectual disabilities were recognised through award of Orders of Australia—Michael Sullivan, Ian Cummins and Fiona McKenzie. Michael's comments at the time capture past problems and challenge all of us to think about our role in bringing about change.

> Every person with an intellectual disability is an individual with a name and a life. We are not just a collection of behaviours or a syndrome full of symptoms. But people with intellectual disabilities are very often treated as if we are nobodies. As if we are invisible ... I want you to ask yourself, 'What could I do, to reach out? What can I do, fix or change, to help someone get the good life they deserve. (https://cid.org.au/our-stories/congratulations-are-in-order/)

This chapter takes up Michael's challenge of making people with intellectual disabilities more visible. It highlights what might be learned by support workers and organisations from listening to what people with intellectual disabilities say about services and suggests some of the actions workers and providers might take to improve or fix some parts of what they do. The chapter includes perspectives of family members as well as of people with intellectual disabilities. This draws attention to the importance of families in the lives of some service users and families' roles as advocates monitoring and collaborating with services to assist people to have the best possible quality of life. Inclusion of family recognises that some people with severe or profound intellectual disabilities are not able to reflect on their own experiences even with the best of support. They will remain invisible unless someone else, like a family member who knows them well and interprets their experiences, advocates for them (Jackson, 2023).

The chapter concentrates on people with intellectual disabilities who use group homes or other forms of supported accommodation services.

Only 4 of the 64 studies about group homes published since 2015 include the perspectives of the people who live in them (Bigby, 2023). This is not always due to disinterest on the part of researchers as much group home research has used observational methods to ensure inclusion of people with severe and profound intellectual disabilities (Mansell, 2011).

Insights from Individuals with Intellectual Disabilities: What the Literature Says

People in group homes whose views were captured in these studies all talked about the importance of the way support workers talked to them. People didn't want to be told what to do or be told off, they wanted to be in control of their own everyday lives and decide what to do for themselves. For example, one of the participants in a UK study said,

> It's like if I say like one thing and they say the other. I just feel like they're telling me, it's hard to explain, it's like if I wanna eat something that's not good and things that aren't proper meals, I feel it isn't really down to them to tell me this. They don't have no right do they, controlling over my life and that I don't really need, I really don't'. (Evans & Gore, 2016, p. 8)

The people in this study did value the support and advice support workers could give but what they thought was most important, was how workers interacted with them in giving advice. One person talked about a staff member they liked as, "good at giving advice, what to do what not to do, advice not telling" (Evans & Gore, 2016, p. 8).

The desire to be in control is echoed among people who have moved from group homes to more independent living. In one study people reflected on their appreciation of having greater choice and control since they had moved.

> You can do what you want, please yourself what you do, be home when you want, you don't have to answer to anyone, you please yourself where you want to go, if you want to go to Melbourne for the day you don't have to ask anyone, if you want to bring someone else, you don't have to ask. (Bigby et al., 2017, p. 312)

People also thought that being known by support workers was important. As this participant in a Dutch study explained about one of his support workers:

> She has been my key support worker right from the start. So, yeah, that is quite a difference. And through that you build something together. You don't have to agree on everything, but you build something together. … You get to know each other; you get to know each other better. She comes to understand me better. That I am emotional at the moment, or glad or happy. She can tell from my face when something is going on. (Giesbers et al., 2018, p. 313)

Having regular support workers and knowing which support worker is coming was important both for people in group homes and for those living in other forms of supported accommodation. As one person said about their team of support workers,

> They help us with the menus, cleaning, cooking, shopping, any appointments and we just lost a really good support worker … there's a bit up and down at the moment, we don't know who is coming and who is not … so it's been really unsettling. … Really they need to ring the day before [tell us] who is going to be on and who's not working. … I think this organisation is not really good enough because we need to know, my housemate and I need to know who is coming. (Bigby et al., 2017, p. 313)

The turnover of support workers means not all workers can know a person well. Careful or deep listening by workers is one way at least of compensating for this. Support workers need to listen as several people getting drop in support said,

> I see, a lot of support workers they've got to listen to you. If they don't listen to you, they're not doing their job properly … Yeah, he does [listen] … I rang him this morning about something. He listened to me on the phone, he rang me back. (Max)

> They [support workers] don't care. … I know that I tell them I want that, they walk away. (Sam) (Ashely et al., 2019, p. 704)

These studies were conducted in the UK, the Netherlands and Australia before the NDIS reforms. They give some indication of what people with intellectual disabilities think is important behaviour for support workers—talking respectfully and listening to them. This might be summarised as being attentive and responsive rather than controlling and dismissive.

The rest of this chapter draws on more recent unpublished data from interviews with people with intellectual disabilities and their families about group home services. These interviews were conducted during 2022 as part of an ongoing longitudinal study of the quality of support in group homes (Bigby et al., 2020). All the names are pseudonyms. These sections take a more in-depth approach and different style from the literature discussed earlier in this chapter. They reflect similar themes to those in the literature and add new ones.

Insights from Recent Interviews with People with Intellectual Disabilities in Group Homes

Support workers carry out a blend of support and caring tasks—skilled support that enables people to be engaged in activities and social relationships—care that meets people's basic needs, such as getting up, showering, dressing, eating and moving from one place to another. What mattered to the people in group homes whom we interviewed was the way staff interacted with them in carrying out these tasks—whether support workers were respectful, and whether they knew about their social connections with family beyond the group home.

Kenneth is a middle-aged man who lives in a group home. He was born with an intellectual disability and has a mobility impairment that causes him pain and requires the support of a walker. Kenneth functions independently in many areas of life with minimal prompting or support from direct staff, but he has difficulty washing and cleaning himself. During a face-to-face interview with Kenneth at his group him, he said, "I need a lot of help in the shower, like with washing myself, personal stuff", he said. Kenneth appeared embarrassed and awkward when he described how difficult it is to wipe his own backside. He is often embarrassed, and even mortified, when new or temporary staff are tasked with helping him in matters of personal care and hygiene, specifically showering and toileting. "I get really", he stammered, trying to find the right words, "when unfamiliar people come in from the agency that don't know me". He lowered his head thoughtfully and continued, "because I don't know them. I'm not trying to be nasty. People at the agency come in and they don't sit down and talk to me. They just start doing their bloody work. Get to know people first before you do the job."

Kenneth's experiences demonstrate the importance of support workers focusing on their relationship with the person they support, rather than always on more concrete tasks. For Kenneth, being treated as an individual and upholding his dignity is central to the support process. Kenneth's concerns underscore the importance of support workers, including those who may be there on a temporary basis, being equipped with the necessary knowledge and skills to provide intimate support in a dignified and respectful manner. This means training on what respect looks like, communicating sensitive and personal issues, identifying and responding to signs of distress and understanding that everyone has preferences that must be respected.

The people with intellectual disabilities we interviewed often gave special attention to family relationships. For Glen, a middle-aged man living in a group home in a country town, his extended family play an essential role in supporting his connections to the world outside his home. Glen takes pride in his family, many of whom live nearby, and he often participates in social events like barbeques and birthday celebrations, which give his life meaning.

Erin is a woman in her late twenties living in a group home in a seaside town. Prior to this, she lived with her mother, as her father died many years ago, and her older brother currently lives interstate. According to Erin, her move to the group home was "a big change in her 29-year-old life", and she has found the adjustment particularly difficult. Even after some time, she still experiences a mix of "nervousness" and "excitement" about the transition. Despite this, her mother has always been and continues to be her closest supporter and confidant. As Erin said, "She's always looking out for me". Since moving out of her mother's home, Erin admitted things "get a bit lonely". More recently, Erin's mother has been experiencing health issues, and despite Erin's best efforts to visit her, the COVID-19 pandemic has made it challenging. "All this lockdown, it's been stressing each other out", Erin revealed.

Erin shared details about her social life both inside and outside her group home, expressing her enjoyment of working at the Red Cross and her mixed experiences with the other residents, saying "I have good days and sour days with them". However, she spoke with evident excitement when recalling how she attended her brother's wedding earlier in the year and her passion for music, inspired by her musically gifted older brother.

Erin's close relationship with her mother plays a critical role in maintaining her emotional wellbeing and providing her with opportunities for social engagement beyond the confines of her daily routine. Further, her family members provide important connections to her past, which gives her a sense of continuity despite the major changes she has experienced since moving into her group home.

For Glen and Erin, living close to family is of utmost importance and enriches their overall quality of life. The significance of family to their emotional wellbeing and in supporting connections to the world outside their home suggests support workers need to know about a person's family, and actively support the role they play in a person's life. Effective person-centred support may involve support workers engaging both an individual and their family to better understand a person's perspectives, needs and goals. In turn, through working collaboratively with support workers, families can help identify the types of activities and social opportunities that are important to individuals and help staff find ways to incorporate these into their daily routines.

Perspectives of Families of People with More Severe and Profound Intellectual Disabilities

Families can be important advocates who safeguard the wellbeing of their relatives by identifying and bringing to the attention of managers neglectful or unprofessional behaviours that impede quality of life or put a person at risk of harm. But as this section illustrates many of the issues they identify are the direct impact of system-wide issues on their relative, such as staff turnover and shortages or adequacy of funding for training.

Jenny and Melissa are identical twins born in Scotland in 1964. Complications surrounding Melissa's birth—an episode of hypoxia (low oxygen)—led to intellectual disability and developmental delays. Jenny remembers living with her sister in the family home during the early years. But then things changed. When they were around five years old, their parents, feeling increasingly overburdened by dealing with Melissa's angry outbursts, decided to transfer her to a specialist hospital for those with intellectual disabilities. Jenny expressed that, in retrospect, she thinks it was a desire for normalcy within the family that prompted her parents' decision. Back in the 1960s, the impulse to institutionalise one's child often reflected a mixture of societal pressure, parental preference and the advice of medical professionals. Jenny reminds me that it was a "whole different ball game back then". To this day, she vividly recalls Melissa at the hospital behind locked doors and the padded rooms that were routinely used to involuntarily seclude patients and force compliance. These days, Melissa is almost 60 and lives in a group home in Victoria, and "life is easier" for her, according to Jenny.

While Jenny derives some peace from the knowledge that things are easier for Melissa now, especially when compared to the harmful effects of institutional life, she continues to worry about Melissa's quality of life in terms of social connections (both within and outside the home), staff interaction and the overall support provided. Jenny asked rhetorically, "[D]oes Melissa suffer, and you don't know about it?". "That's always on the back of your mind", she said.

One afternoon, at the height of the COVID-19 pandemic, Jenny received a call from a support worker at Melissa's group home to inform her that her sister had been rushed to hospital in an ambulance after having a seizure. Jenny arrived at the hospital shortly thereafter to find Melissa in the isolation ward for COVID patients. Melissa was under-dressed in soiled pyjamas, according to Jenny, her hair in a multitude of knots, "in a state of neglect", as she put it. She'd vomited and nobody had bothered to change her. A nurse commented, "My God, her hair hasn't been brushed for days", Jenny recalls. The remark stung, especially since Jenny, and her parents before her, has always taken pride in making sure Melissa's hair is done nicely and that she is dressed well. For Jenny, a respectable appearance projects a message of dignity.

When Jenny inquired about what had happened leading up to her sister's hospitalisation, the support workers from Melissa's group home were not forthcoming with the details. In fact, Jenny found unsettling discrepancies between what the support workers said and what she uncovered through her own investigation. For example, according to Jenny, the ambulance had not been called until an hour after the time she'd been given. Furthermore, no one was able to tell her what had happened between the time Melissa received her morning medication and when the ambulance was called a couple of hours later. "We don't know the truth of what happened that morning", Jenny said. "And I don't think they [service provider representatives] are prepared to actually be an open book with us". Without all the details, Jenny was left to piece together the story herself. She believes the direct support worker on shift that morning suspected Melissa of having COVID and therefore quarantined her in her bedroom, neglecting to take proper care of her from fear of infection. Jenny explained, "We think they have given Melissa her tablets, not made her sit up to take them, but given them to her while she's still in bed, and she's probably choked on them and vomited, and then had a seizure". Then, after a long pause, she said, "[W]e don't know".

Jenny's experience with her sister's hospitalisation highlights the complex challenges that service providers and support workers face in their work. It highlights the need for transparency in communications with individuals and families. If errors were made, Jenny wanted these to be acknowledged and disclosed—a principle known as "open disclosure" (Iedema et al., 2008). The story of Melissa and Jenny highlights the essential role of family connections in advocating for individuals who cannot speak up for themselves and the necessity for ties to people outside the service system for safeguarding the rights and wellbeing of people with disabilities.

"You worry all the time": The Impact of Staff Turnover and Leadership

Like Jenny in the previous section, one father, Gerald, echoed similar concerns about a lack of transparency and communication in relation to the support of his 38-year-old daughter, Julie, who also lives in a group home in Victoria. "There's always things you worry and ponder about", he said. "Does she get a good level of care or is it that when you turn away the carers [staff] don't do what they appear to be doing when you're there. You worry all the time." Since her mother's health began to wane, Gerald has become Julie's primary advocate and confidant. He admits that Julie sometimes calls him to tell him she does not feel safe when there are new or temporary support staff around. Because of this, he frequently spends weekend evenings at Julie's group home to provide her comfort and "monitor things", as he puts it. Sadly, what he sees there gives him little respite from his worries. He is often struck by the high levels of disengagement among staff. People "wasting time", he said, watching TV or playing on their phones, rather than being attentive and responsive to the people around them. He expressed caution about asserting himself to the staff from fear they might find him "too demanding" and of there "being a backlash" against his daughter.

Gerald's depiction of Julie's discomfort around new or temporary direct support staff strikes a chord with other individuals residing in group homes, such as Kenneth, whose account we previously heard with relation to dignified support. Gerald's concerns about Julie's support reflect a range of quality of life domains. He worries about her physical safety and emotional wellbeing when she is with unfamiliar staff members. Additionally, he feels guilty about the limited opportunities for Julie to participate in social activities and form meaningful relationships. Although Julie enjoys socialising, she cannot entertain herself and often spends lengthy periods alone with few activities or opportunities for her to receive the warmth, affection and closeness related to the quality of interpersonal relationships. As Gerald explained, rarely do they [staff] engage her more fully in extended conversation because "that's what she likes, that's her strength".

Gerald believes that if staff members took the time to engage Julie in conversation, it would enhance her sense of wellbeing. Unfortunately, he says they rarely take the time to talk with her at length, which leads Julie to call him multiple times per evening for someone to talk to. However, when she has a one-on-one support worker he doesn't hear from her as often. "Then it's okay", he said, "she's good". During these times he feels reassured that she is receiving the attention and engagement she needs.

Gerald feels a strong sense of disempowerment over the lack of consistent strong leadership at Julie's group home. According to him, the home hasn't "had a regular manager for five to eight years", and there's always someone temporary who stays for a few months before leaving. "If there was stability in that regard", he explained, "as a parent, you would go away feeling far more confident". Strong leadership is crucial because it influences how support is enacted, and for many families, this is of utmost importance. As one mother said, referring to the care of her middle-aged son, "When he has had a long-term team leader, and they get to know him, they do start caring a little bit and they investigate more options for him. They involve themselves more in the activities he likes." Similarly, Jenny attributed the lack of transparency and accountability she has experienced to a lack of strong and consistent leadership and high staff turnover at Melissa's group home. "They need one person in there who knows what's happening", she said. In the past, when there was staff stability, the communication was better, giving her "more faith" in the support being provided to Melissa.

Gerald likened the lack of strong leadership to a boat without a captain. "It's a bit like a boat in the middle of the ocean", he said. "If you've got a captain in charge, you may get to port. If you don't, the chance of getting to port are pretty slim." He continued, "I think the whole house can feel it as well, in the sense of there's no spontaneity, no natural happiness". In Julie's case, he hopes that with strong management in the future things will turn around at her group home. Currently, there is a young woman temporarily managing things that sets him at ease. He described her as "very understanding of Julie" and as someone who is "not scared to initiate contact" with him. "She keeps the place running pretty well", he said, adding that when he is there he can see "she knows what is going on, she knows what to do, and she directs the other staff accordingly". "A good manager solves eighty percent of the problems", Gerald explained, because they "monitor the situation carefully in terms of what the staff do, they make sure they [direct support staff] get proper training, and make sure they know each individual client and what their needs and requirements are". Gerald's awareness of the gold standards for frontline managers that enable best practice and lead to quality outcomes for people in group homes is consistent with evidence-based best practice frameworks (Bigby, 2023).

Given that the disability sector reports high rates of staff turnover and that providers are reporting increasing difficulty attracting team leaders and house managers, there are no simple solutions to the frustration experienced by Gerald and many parents. Support workers and providers can demonstrate empathy for the frustration and disappointment experienced by people supported and their families about the high rates of turnover. Providers should do what they can to improve the attraction and retention of staff. Providers might focus on more than the team leader or manager, and think about how selected team members—or even all team members—could learn about the person supported. Providers should design their systems to enable new managers and workers to quickly understand the wants and needs of each person supported and to minimise the need for the people supported or families to have to repeat themselves time and time again, which can be both frustrating and demoralising. For example, short videos can be recorded conveying the key information about the person and how best to support them.

Rosemarie, a divorced mother of four children in her sixties is continually frustrated about the quality of support her middle-aged son, Tom, receives in his group home. She feels perpetually exhausted from continually monitoring the support he receives and responding to incidents that result from staff practices. "I am constantly involved", she said. "Constantly." Recently, Tom got into a fist fight with another resident from his group home on the bus as they were coming home from their day programmes. "Andrew, who lives with Tom, makes noises", Rosemarie explained, "and it gets on Tom's nerves". Tom turned around and "whopped him one" and "told him to shut up". In retaliation Andrew slapped Tom across the face, and then "it was on for young and old", Rosemarie explained. For Rosemarie, the most concerning thing about the incident was that it could have been avoided. She explained that the staff and residents are aware of the tension that exists between Tom and Andrew, so "why was Tom sitting in front of Andrew on the bus?" "Stuff-ups happen all the time", she said, giving in to her frustration, before adding offhandedly that "it's not great when they ring you up and tell you they've lost him".

Rosemarie wrote a letter of complaint to the current team manager of Tom's group home about the staff's practices and management of the situation on the bus and the dismal implementation of her son's behaviour support plan, but it was clear that she lacked any hope of reaching a satisfying resolution. Rosemarie's frustration over staff competence and frequent episodes of "negligence" has reached an intolerable point for her, which is further exacerbated by staff turnover and her consequent inability to form a strong working relationship with a long-term team leader who might meet the profound need for staff training and development. "If they would stay in their role for any period of time, then I would have some sort of relationship", she said.

Support staff and managers interacting with Rosemarie and other family members like her should recognise that their frustration often results from years of disappointments. Confronting years of pent-up frustration can make staff feel anxious or defensive. One way of reducing the impact in Rosemarie's case would be support workers and managers focussing on the present and demonstrating that good support to Tom is possible through evidence informed practice such as Active Support. Further, a service manager might acknowledge to her the reasons behind people such as Tom and Andrew, who though incompatible, might have had to live together. When in the past for example, places in group homes were scarce and avoiding homelessness in a crisis rather than compatibility was the driving force for filling vacancies. A manager might also initiate discussion about the greater opportunities that individualised funding brings in terms of exploring alternatives to good groups or reconfiguring existing support arrangements.

Through listening to individuals and families, support staff may also identify "bigger" issues of concern such in the case of Erin and Rosemarie compatibility with the people they live with or indeed where a person lives. In fact, several people who were interviewed expressed a desire to live somewhere closer to shops where they could walk and get coffee, and for those already near shops and places to go out, it was a factor in their satisfaction with their living situation. Although often beyond the influence of a support worker, insights into concerns such as these should not be dismissed as too hard to fix but be passed on managers or support coordinators who can support people to act on them.

Communication Between Families, Staff and the People They Support

Social engagement is a crucial aspect of life for individuals with disabilities living in group homes. However, families often express concerns about their relative's limited social networks and believe that support workers can play a role in providing social opportunities. As one mother, speaking about her son's support, put it, "I would like him to achieve as much socialisation as possible in the community, to be able to perhaps even find some volunteering job that he would like to do, say, at Bunnings or Safeway or something like that. But he needs to be supported in that."

Families hope that staff can prioritise getting to know their family members as unique individuals with distinct personalities, interests, feelings and idiosyncrasies. This they surmise will lead to effective support for engagement in social activities that broaden and strengthen social networks.

The importance of personalised attention and support can be seen in the case of Jenny and her twin sister, Melissa, where staff turnover and absenteeism have made it challenging for staff to provide the consistency in support that lends itself to rapport building and responsiveness, as Jenny explained. "Lately, they've had a lot of changes in the staff", she shared with me. Although some staff members developed strong relationships with Melissa in the past, they had since moved on. "This is the problem that you have", Jenny said. "People have lives outside. It's just their job."

Because Melissa is non-verbal, Jenny has taken it upon herself to educate support staff and team leaders about her sister's likes and dislikes regarding food, music, games and more, and has even created visual slideshows containing essential information about Melissa to enhance staff learning. As Jenny said, "It takes time to get to know somebody, and every individual person with a disability is different".

She elaborated on Melissa's particular sensitivity to certain sounds and her fondness for certain pet names. "When we argue or if somebody is noisy", Jenny explained, "Melissa thinks that's quite funny. She gets stimulated from that." She continued by saying, "We call her a nick name that she thinks it's hilarious. So, we've told her support workers to call her that." Jenny is aware that temporary staff covering a shift may not have the luxury of reviewing copious amounts of paperwork. Thus, she hopes the slideshow will offer a more user-friendly, time-efficient and concise alternative to enhance the quality of Melissa's support. While acknowledging the challenges faced by support staff, it's important to ensure that residents receive individualised support that meets their specific needs.

One way to overcome these challenges to delivering person-centred support is through improved communication between people supported, families and group home staff. By sharing important information about their loved one's likes, dislikes and preferences, families can help staff provide personalised support that promotes social engagement and meaningful activities. Families can also complement the role of staff by building relationships and providing ideas for meaningful activities. Effective collaboration between families and group home staff is essential to achieve better support and quality of life outcomes for individuals with disabilities. However, even with the best intentions and efforts towards personalised support, communication breakdown between families and service providers can hinder the progress and positive outcomes for individuals with disabilities.

This can be seen in the case of Kerry, who has taken on a larger role in managing the support of her younger sister, Catherine, who lives in a group home in Victoria. With both sisters in their fifties, Kerry has slowly taken the lead in managing Catherine's support as their parents have stepped back. Kerry's experience highlights the need for good communication, including good listening, by workers. Despite her efforts to communicate her sister's preferences and needs, Kerry states that her contributions are often overlooked or disregarded by staff, and this undermines an effective working relationship between them.

For example, Kerry shared that as a source of comfort and joy for her sister, she often buys DVDs of the TV comedy *The Golden Girls*, which has always been one of Catherine's favourite shows. Recently, after a conversation with support staff, Kerry decided to purchase a smart TV for Catherine's bedroom, with the intention of not only allowing her to stream her beloved show, but also providing her with the added possibility of accessing new content.

"We thought it was a great idea for her birthday", Kerry said. "So mum, dad, and I went halves in it, but also too in the hope that she might watch something else if she had the opportunity to look through [new content]." However, despite Kerry's clear intention, a new team leader soon reached out to request more DVDs for Catherine, as her previous one's had gone missing.

In Kerry's case, the purchase of the smart TV was intended to broaden Catherine's viewing options and expose her to new content. For Kerry, the team leader's response not only indicated a breakdown in communication but also a misalignment in their goals and values for creating new opportunities for Catherine.

While the frustration of the family is understandable, even small changes need to be carefully communicated and managed by both staff and family. In Catherine's case, it may have been necessary for;

- The family to convey their intentions to Catherine, explaining the perceived advantage of being able to watch new content.
- The family to discuss their goal with the team leader, who can convey this to the team.
- The team leader to check with Catherine and members of the support worker team whether they know how to operate a smart TV. If not, training would be needed.
- To arrange some training for Catherine about using the smart TV, such as a video of the steps for turning it on and finding channels or a guide in Easy Read.
- To arrange some training for staff in how to use the smart TV that could be recorded and available to any new or casual staff.
- Regular communication between the team leader and Kerry about the progress that has been made, and barriers that may need to be addressed.

Indeed, Kerry spoke of other events that have pointed to a similar misalignment in goals regarding Catherine's support. For example, a couple of years ago Kerry suggested they spend some of Catherine's NDIS funding for one-on-one support and try out a hot springs facility as an alternative water-based experience for Catherine, who loves swimming and water play.

Again, Kerry hoped the suggestion would enable Catherine to try something new, deviating from her usual routine of swimming at the local pool. However, her suggestion faced resistance, and the priority of returning home at an established hour took precedence over creating a new experience for Catherine. This indicated to Kerry the team at the house were not fully committed to broadening Catherine's experiences beyond her usual routine. "I don't understand why it was an issue", she said. Such challenges emphasise the need for effective communication and collaboration between families and service providers to ensure the best possible outcomes for individuals with disabilities.

This example might be considered as a micro-change that requires good communication to make it successful. The team leader would need to:

- Communicate to Catherine about the proposed change and seek her views.
- Assess any risks at the hot springs facility and if necessary make changes in staff rosters and the ratio of support workers.
- Review the current contract of support, and whether additional funding is required.
- Communicate to staff team members about the new arrangements and that the usual return time is no longer required.
- If staff want to return home to the group home at the established hour, explore reasons for this (which might be appropriate or inappropriate) and how those concerns might be remedied.
- Communication by the team leader back to Kerry.

Many people supported, families and support workers share values aligned with the primary principles of the NDIS, such a choice and control, and the broadening of experiences to improve quality of life for the person being supported. Where values are aligned but things still go wrong, the remedies might be found in improved communication and the appropriate management of micro-change.

Effective leadership at the frontline is critical in shaping the culture of group homes, and the values and attitudes of team leaders can have a significant impact on the people being supported. Families recognise this impact and have shared their experiences, with some highlighting inadequate leadership resulting in negative outcomes, while others have praised positive attitudes and behaviours improving the quality of their relative's wellbeing. One sister, commenting on the team leader who oversees her brother's group home, said, "I love her energy and her passion for people with a disability. I mean, she's close to them. They relate to her. She talks to them. You can have a person who has all the administrative skills in the world and that can run a house efficiently, but if they don't have the passion and pull, they'll never warm to her."

However, communication breakdowns arising from staff instability, a lack of strong leadership and a mismatch in values and objectives between families and service providers can leave individuals feeling unsupported and unheard. Group homes that foster a culture of support and recognise the distinct viewpoints of families can facilitate successful working relationships between service providers and families, ultimately improving the quality of life for those with disabilities.

Conclusions

For people with intellectual disabilities, such as Kenneth and those mentioned in the introduction, the way in which support and personal care are provided is just as important as what is provided. Support workers and managers must always give attention to how the interaction with people, to building relationships and enabling people to feel at ease.

For Jenny, Gerald and Rosemarie, as family members, strong team leadership can help embed a culture of accountability and enable constructive collaboration between families and service providers. By establishing clear expectations and regular communication channels, a more open dialogue can be created to ensure the individual with disability's needs and preferences are being met. This type of constructive relationship can help prevent conflicts (not disagreements) and instead lead to effective communication aimed at improving the individual's life (Mayer, 2009). Indeed, as has been reported, some family members praised positive attitudes and pointed to the behaviours of team leaders that improved the quality of their relative's wellbeing.

Person-centred Active Support and Frontline Practice Leadership are identified as key evidence informed practices that improve quality of life for individuals in group homes (Bigby, 2023). The experiences shared by individuals with disabilities and families in this chapter can also provide valuable guidance for practitioners and managers in the disability sector, highlighting the need for collaborative and person-centred support.

It is crucial to recognise the importance of centring the voices of people with disabilities in identifying their support needs and preferences. By considering the perceptions and understandings of individuals with disabilities and their families, practitioners can gain a more holistic understanding of a person's needs and preferences.

First, service providers should prioritise effective communication with individuals with disabilities and their families to establish an open dialogue about mutual expectations, needs and concerns. This requires clear and transparent communication channels, regular updates and a willingness to listen and respond to feedback.

Second, service providers should promote a culture of accountability and teamwork, through strong Frontline Practice Leadership and training that equips staff with the skills they need. Training programmes should prioritise skills in providing sensitive personal care, and supporting communication, choice and engagement of the people they support through staff use of Active Support, as well as empathy and strategies for collaborating with families.

Third, service providers should support the maintenance of family relationships where appropriate, recognising the value of diverse perspectives in decision-making and support planning processes. This can help gain a more holistic view of a person's needs and preferences and help in working together to provide person-centred support that enhances the quality of life and wellbeing for people with disabilities.

Fourth, service providers should enable people with disabilities to expand their social connections by engaging them in activities that align with their interests, foster regular community involvement and facilitate meaningful social interactions within the local community. To enable effective support and engagement in social activities that broaden and strengthen social networks, service providers should prioritise getting to know the person on an individual basis.

Overall, by adopting these strategies and working closely with individuals with disabilities and families, service providers can promote better quality of life and meet the diverse support needs of people in group homes while honouring their voices and individuality.

Take Home Messages

- Ensuring that the "voice" of the person being supported is heard is fundamental to good quality support. For those who cannot express their needs and preferences, every attempt must be made to interpret their will and preferences.
- Usually, family and other supporters are allies in providing good quality support. Team members should seek sound relationships with families and other supporters.
- Encourage open disclosure: acknowledging and disclosing errors helps maintain trust and promotes the rights and wellbeing of individuals with disabilities.
- Consistent leadership and staff retention strategies are key to empowering families and ensuring the wellbeing of individuals in group homes.
- Support for engagement in activities and respectful conversations significantly enhance residents' wellbeing and satisfaction with support.
- Innovative tools, such as short videos, can help convey important information about residents, enabling new staff to quickly understand and support the person effectively.

References

Ashley, D., Fossey, E., & Bigby, C. (2019). The home environments and occupational engagements of people with intellectual disabilities in supported living: "It's been better than the last place I lived". *British Journal of Occupational Therapy, 82*, 688–709. https://doi.org/10.1177/0308022619843080

Bigby, C. (2023). Evidence about best practice in supported accommodation services: What needs to be in place. NDIS Quality and Safeguarding Commission. https://www.ndiscommission.gov.au/resources/reports-policies-and-frameworks/inquiries-and-reviews/own-motion-inquiry-aspects and Living with Disability Research Centre, La Trobe University https://doi.org/10.26181/21769067

Bigby, C., Bould, E., & Beadle-Brown, J. (2017). Conundrums of supported living: The experiences of people with intellectual disability. *Journal of Intellectual & Developmental Disability, 42*(4), 309–319. https://doi.org/10.3109/13668250.2016.1253051

Bigby, C., Bould, E., Iacono, I., & Beadle-Brown, J. (2020). Predicting good active support for people with intellectual disabilities in supported accommodation services: Key messages for providers, consumers and regulators. *Journal of Intellectual and Developmental Disability.*, *45*, 279–289. https://doi.org/10.3109/13668250.2019.1685479

Evans, T., & Gore, N. (2016). Staff behaviours valued by service users: Views of people whose behaviour challenges. *International Journal of Positive Behavioural Support, 6*(2) Autumn 2016, 4–11.

Giesbers, S. A. H., Hendriks, L., Jahoda, A., Hastings, R. P., & Embregts, P. J. C. M. (2018). Living with support: Experiences of people with mild intellectual disability. *Journal of Applied Research in Intellectual Disabilities, 32*, 446–456. https://doi.org/10.1111/jar.12542

Iedema, R., Sorensen, R., Manias, E., Tuckett, A., Piper, D., Mallock, N., Williams, A., & Jorm, C. (2008). Patients' and family members' experiences of open disclosure following adverse events. *International Journal for Quality in Health Care, 20*, 421–432. https://doi.org/10.1093/intqhc/mzn043)

Jackson, A. J. (2023). Between us: Facilitated decision-making in the relational experience of profound intellectual disability Abstract Ethos. https://doi.org/10.1111/etho.12406

Mansell, J. (2011). *Structured observational research in services for people with learning disabilities*. Methods Review. School for Social Research.

Mayer, B. (2009). *Staying with Conflict: A strategic approach to ongoing disputes*. Jossey-Bass.

CHAPTER 4

Supporting Community Participation

Christine Bigby

Community participation is a difficult concept to pin down. It takes many forms—going out with friends to an exhibition, the cinema or for lunch; playing sport; volunteering in a charity shop or coaching the local football team; attending a cooking class at a neighbourhood house; being a member of a walking club; or simply regularly going to the local swimming pool. It means being engaged in an activity and most likely some form of social interaction with others be they strangers, peers, friends or people who recognise you as another club member or participant. Community participation is the type of thing that is often taken for granted as part of everyday life. What it looks like depends on an individual's preferences, available resources and opportunities in their environment. Despite its everyday nature, community participation is a key objective of disability policy. This is illustrated in the objectives of the Australian National Disability Insurance Scheme Act (2013) which include:

- to support the independence and social and economic participation of people with disability;

C. Bigby (✉)
Living with Disability Research Centre, La Trobe University, Melbourne, VIC, Australia
e-mail: C.Bigby@latrobe.edu.au

C. Bigby, A. Hough (eds.), *Disability Practice*,
https://doi.org/10.1007/978-981-99-6143-6_4

- to promote the provision of high-quality and innovative supports that enable people with disability to maximise independent lifestyles and full inclusion in the community; and
- to raise community awareness of the issues that affect the social and economic participation of people with disability and facilitate greater community inclusion of people with disability.

Support for community participation is also central to Australia's National Disability Strategy 2021–2031. Policy Priority 3 of the Strategy states that:

> People with disability should be supported to live more accessible and connected lives within their communities, including being able to fully participate in social, recreational, sporting, religious and cultural life. (p. 11)

Policy wording is often inexact, using words such as *community* and *social*, or *inclusion* and *participation* interchangeably. Disability services sometimes using terms such as *accessing the community* which distances community participation from everyday life. How many people without disabilities refer to going to a yoga class for example as 'community access'? Since the 1980s, significant government funding has been invested in supporting community participation; indeed, with the advent of the NDIS in Australia, more than 72% of adults with disabilities and 76% of those with intellectual disability who are NDIS participants were funded to realise goals for community participation in their plans (NDIA, 2022, p. 184).

The first part of this chapter explores the reasons why community participation is such an important part of disability policy and expenditure. It describes the low levels of community participation among people with intellectual disabilities, identifies the obstacles in their way and explains its significance to a good quality of life. The chapter then examines different ways of conceptualising community participation, the role of service providers and synthesises evidence about effective programs and practice into a practice framework to inform action. The final section considers strategies beyond individuals for maximising social participation of people with intellectual disabilities in their communities of choice.

Why Support for Community Participation Is Important

People with intellectual disabilities are considerably disadvantaged in terms of community participation compared to some other disability groups and the general population. Therefore, this chapter concentrates on people whose primary disability is an intellectual one, although some of the strategies discussed apply to other groups such as people with psychosocial disabilities.

People with intellectual disabilities have been framed as being 'present rather than participating' in communities and as 'living in a distinct social space' made up of family, people with disabilities and paid staff (Clement & Bigby, 2010). Evidence shows they are more likely to be lonely, socially isolated, disconnected from their locality and dissatisfied with neighbours or local community. They are less likely to be members of community groups, to go out, see friends or be engaged in activities or social interactions when they do go out (AIHW, 2022). One of the reasons for this is that people with intellectual disabilities experience many of the circumstances that limit or obstruct participation—they are likely to have smaller social networks, fewer friends and are often reliant on paid staff for support. They are more likely to have a low income, experience difficulties with transport and getting to and from places and have an increased likelihood of experiencing unwelcoming attitudes and discrimination from others. All of these factors mean that people with intellectual disabilities are likely to require support to select and participate in communities of their choice; there is also a need for broader social change to address the attitudinal and structural obstacles to their participation.

The following first-hand accounts from research exploring community participation illustrate the breadth of experiences it encompasses, and the enjoyment that goes with it (Bigby, et al. 2018a).

> Talking about the gig buddy program she is part of Sue said "I feel like I can be myself. And have fun and go out and that. So, I'm not with Mum and Dad all the time. ... I always wanted to have a friend to hang out with and do things with and enjoy the world out there." Another participant Mel said, "I like the fact that we are able to go out in the evenings and socialise and everything. And just able to have fun with our buddies. And get to know each other. I'm going to a Christmas party on Friday night with my gig buddy so we're going to meet up and go to the city."

> Talking about the Arts program she attends several days a week, Elizabeth said, "I've got good friends here and we all love doing our art. They are very understanding of my problems. I feel comfortable." John who also goes to the program said, "I am an artist. People like my stuff. They buy my stuff… it's a better place than other places I've been in the past. Now I am an artist."

> Talking about the football club he belongs to, a member said, "I just like coming out. Sunday, kicking the footy. That's what it's all about."

Research suggests that some staff in disability services think it is unrealistic to expect people with more severe intellectual disabilities to participate in communities and at best they may be able to be present in communities (Clement & Bigby, 2010). This research shows, for example, that often people living in group homes are taken out *into the community* in groups or alone with a staff member without real purpose, do not interact with anyone but staff and are not engaged in any activities. As one support worker said about community participation, 'It's pretty hard with our ones, they can't talk, the more able bodied can participate' (Bigby et al., 2009, p. 363). One way of changing such attitudes and practices is to demonstrate that everyone can participate with the right support, no matter how severe their disability. This is illustrated in the following excerpts that describe participation by people with severe disabilities who don't use language.

> James, a support worker, described the experience of a person he supported where "one day of the week he spends time volunteering and assisting at the SES, he might do things like washing trucks which is a job that would need to be done by someone else so it's significant, it's important, absolutely … he's got his SES kind of jacket on which is one of those fluoro outfits … he understands that yes he is volunteering, he is working as part of the SES volunteer cohort and there are many people who volunteer as part of the SES, he's no different in that respect." (Bigby, et al. 2018a)
>
> Trudi, a support worker, talked with Chloe about her weekly participation at a local swimming pool: "you meet Jim when you first get there. He does an exercise program at the pool nearly every day. You'll take his hand sometimes, Chloe, and you'll go and walk the length of the pool with him. She went on to say that Chloe had another gentleman that she sees there, Robin, who she has formed a great friendship with. And she will actually wait and knows about roughly what time he gets there and she'll be watching to see." (Bigby, et al. 2018a)

Experiences of community participation contribute to having a good quality of life. Despite its different forms, when people are participating in the way they choose they are likely to experience increased self-esteem, confidence, wider social networks, improved skills and better health. As community participation often means that others outside their immediate service are involved in a person's life or see them regularly, it can also act as a safeguard against abuse or exploitation.

Understanding Community Participation

In the 1970s normalisation was the dominant ideology in disability services. It meant community participation was often understood as participating in valued social activities, having firm relationships with people without disabilities and using mainstream or non-segregated places that were open to everyone. Since then, dogmatic certainty about the types of activities, people and places that should constitute community participation has disappeared. It has become clear that mainstream places are not always welcoming. Indeed, recent research shows that choices by people with intellectual disabilities about where to go are often based on factors other than whether a place is mainstream, and instead include familiarity, the quality or type of activities on offer or existing relationships with the people there (Wiesel et al., 2022).

An overarching definition of community participation is the "performance of people in actual activities in social life domains through interaction with others in the context in which they live" (Verdonschot et al., 2009). This way of seeing community participation is derived from the World Health Organisation's International Classification of Functioning, Disability and Health (ICF) framework. It suggests that community participation has three essential elements: *activities*, *social interactions* and *place*. That is, doing something, somewhere, that involves interaction with others. This definition is not prescriptive about the types of activities, people or places that constitute community participation but rather recognises that every person has their own preferences about the type of community participation they enjoy or want to experience. Individual choice is important, recognising that:

- friendships or shared activities with peers with disabilities rather than people without disabilities may be preferred sometimes by some people;

- community has diverse meanings and is not necessarily a neighbourhood or locality but may be a group of people with shared interests such as hikers or with shared identities such as the lesbian, gay, bisexual, transgender and intersexed communities;
- subjective feelings such as belonging or conviviality are important to some people; and
- relationships other than friendships, such as being recognised by other participants as a regular member of a yoga class, can lead to positive social interactions (Bigby & Wiesel, 2019).

Although the nature of community participation is diverse, having a shared language to talk about it and an understanding of its essential elements is important to delivering effective support. Shared language and understanding of community participation helps support workers and service providers to articulate their aims: what type of support they should provide a person, and how to design programs that draw on effective strategies or skills. Shared language and understanding also helps people with intellectual disabilities and those who support them—such as families or support coordinators—to be effective consumers by knowing what options are available to choose from and the type of support or community participation they prefer. Finally, shared understandings of community participation are important to ensuring accountability for government funds, enabling the development of criteria about the nature and quality of what is purchased, and the outcomes achieved for individuals.

Supporting Community Participation

The very nature of intellectual disability means that people are likely to require support with making decisions about the type of community participation they prefer, exploring options, negotiating access, getting to places, participating in activities and interacting with others and their environment when they get there. The type, timing and longevity of support needed depend on each individual and their circumstances. Others in the community without intellectual disabilities are also likely to require support to be welcoming, to communicate with and to understand how to include a person with intellectual disability in their group or facility. These other community members are often referred to as natural supporters (Bigby & Anderson, 2021).

Traditionally, support for community participation was provided through offsite activities offered by day centres, day programs, leisure programs or by staff in the case of those living in group homes. Although some programs offered tailored opportunities and support to individuals, the type and quality of support varied (Bigby, 2005). Too often in day programs support for community participation was muddled together with ensuring a person had somewhere to go during the day if they were unsafe to be at home alone.

In Australia, and internationally, much has changed as a result of the shift to individualised funding: some day programs have closed, and others have reinvented themselves as community hubs offering individualised support for participation. Others have created social enterprises that provide opportunities for volunteer work or interactions with community members. Innovative programs have taken new approaches such as recruiting and training volunteers or bringing together peers with common interests, and attention has been given to making mainstream facilities and programs more inclusive.

In Australia, with the establishment of the NDIS, more choice is now available to people with intellectual disabilities to support community participation. As well as using service providers, there are options for people or their families to employ their own workers to support community participation. Effective support for community participation however is much more than the *frontstage* or visible, direct one-to-one support; it requires supporters to have skills, knowledge and time to do the *backstage* or behind-the-scenes work. As the next sections explain, community participation is more than going out into the *community* with a support worker acting as a paid companion. Much depends on where people go, how regularly and accessing the quality of support needed to be engaged in an activity or social interactions when they get there. This is the *backstage* work to support community participation and, if it is done well, over time natural supporters may replace some, or all, of the role support workers play.

Program Design and Practice for Supporting Community Participation

For some people, families or other allies may plan and oversee the backstage work that facilitates community participation. They may also supervise the frontstage work by hiring and monitoring the work of supporter workers and ensuring support workers are skilled. Most people however will rely on programs delivered by service providers to do both backstage and frontstage work. This section describes the design of different types of community participation programs that research suggests are effective and lead to good quality of life outcomes for the people they support. Describing different types of programs helps to illustrate the backstage, often invisible, work of supporting community participation. Programs provide the infrastructure that enables individuals to make choices and receive effective individualised support; very few remain that operate on the type of group mentality of the past where people were offered a limited menu of choices and most things happened in groups necessitated by funding rather than participant choice.

The design of programs and the interventions or strategies to support community participation can be quite different, as they emphasise different aspects of participation (Bigby, et al. 2018 b). Knowing the different aspects of community participation that programs might emphasise helps a person to think more about what they want from participation and to choose what type of program they prefer. It also helps to guide the type of support a worker provides. The following examples help illustrate the different aspects of community participation that programs emphasise and types of programs this leads to.

Emphasising Social Relationships

Having social relationships with others who are not paid workers increases opportunities for a person to interact socially and participate in a range of activities and community groups. If a program emphasises relationships, then strategies focus on developing new social relationships by matching a person with a volunteer or helping a person find places or activities where they might meet others with similar interests. For example, in the earlier excerpt, the gig buddy program assisted Sue to build a friendship with a volunteer and have someone to go to gigs with.

Programs that Build Social Relationships

These types of programs aim to match participants with volunteers who have similar interests to their own, providing opportunities for shared activities and friendship. Staff work at getting to know participants, learning about things such as their interests, personality, where they live, age and skills by talking to them and those who know them well. Such information is important in matching them with a volunteer who they get on with and who lives in a similar locality. Programs promote their aims and recruit volunteers through various forms of advertising and websites that act as clearing houses for those seeking to volunteer. Before volunteers are accepted into a program, they are usually vetted by requiring, for example, a NDIS screening and police check, or providing referees and having an interview with staff. Once accepted volunteers receive some form of training. This might include briefing about the program, the expectations of volunteers such as the number of hours they spend with their matched participant each month, the code of conduct and background information about disability policies and safeguarding requirements. Training might also include tips about beginning relationships, communication and managing common issues identified as arising in programs, such as the difference between friendship and support work.

Once training is completed staff discuss the match with both the volunteer and the participant and introduce them, often facilitating their first meeting. The matched pair are left to organise future meetings around mutually chosen activities. These may be going to sports events, concerts, cinemas, restaurants or sharing time together with others in their network in private homes. Program staff remain available to mentor either volunteers or participants should problems or queries arise. Some programs organise activities for small groups such as dinner or going to a gig, to offer opportunities for participants who are waiting for a match, as well as matched pairs. They may use newsletters to keep people in touch with the program and share information about upcoming events or discounts that may have been negotiated. For more detailed information see descriptions of a Gig Buddy Program (Bigby, et al. 2018a) and a Leisure Buddy program (Fyffe & Raskin, 2015). Volunteer programs such as these primarily include people with relatively low support needs often excluding people with more severe disabilities. As one staff member from a Gig Buddy program said:

> In an ideal world you would include everybody, and there have been times where we've had to say if there's no communication, it makes it really hard. Because one thing we say to volunteers is we don't ever want you to be a support worker, because that changes the relationship. (Bigby, et al. 2018a, p. 61)

The balance of participants to volunteers in programs is often uneven meaning people may wait for a long time; and in large cities distances between where people live can make matches difficult. The point where people become friends, rather than participants and volunteers, is ill-defined which may raise issues around safeguarding if backup support from the program ceases.

Some befriending programs may be less formal and more inclusive of people with more severe intellectual disabilities. Their focus may be on staff nurturing a potential friendship a staff member might have identified or supporting a person to find and participate in activities where they are likely to meet someone who over time may become a friend (Amado, 2014).

Emphasising Pleasant Social Interactions or Convivial Encounters

Sharing an activity or identity with others in places such as libraries, community groups or volunteer organisations leads to pleasant social interactions which if they happen regularly mean a person becomes recognised and known by others. Although valued for themselves, over time convivial encounters may become firmer relationships or friendships. If a program emphasises convivial encounters strategies focus on finding community groups or public facilities which provide opportunities to share an activity and interact with other people. For example, in the earlier excerpt, going regularly to the local swimming pool meant Chloe was recognised and greeted by other regular swimmers who smiled at her and over time learned her name.

Programs that Create and Support Opportunities for Convivial Encounters

These types of programs aim to create and support opportunities for a person to regularly share activities with others and engage in friendly or convivial social interactions. Convivial encounters take place in community groups or classes, public facilities such as libraries or commercial places such as leisure centres. They involve interaction between people with and without intellectual disabilities and, though friendly, are not friendships as there is no expected contact outside the context in which the encounter occurs unless two people serendipitously see each other.

Programs may be called community options, community access or volunteering and are offered as part of day programs, community hubs or retirement programs for people with intellectual disabilities. Programs usually serve 20 or more participants. However, what they offer each person is individualised although the person may not always participate in activities on their own. To illustrate this, Table 4.1 summarises different examples of convivial encounters and strategies for creating them. As Table 4.1 shows, plans need to be made at the program level to create opportunities that are tailored either to an individual or small group of participants. As with programs that assist in building relationships programs, staff also plan with each individual to understand their skills, support needs and interests.

Once activities such as those in Table 4.1 are identified or created, staff begin a process of matching and introducing the participant. This requires staff knowledge of the person from the planning process and knowledge about community groups, places and task analysis. For example, staff need to understand whether the place or group will be a good match for the person by understanding its culture and rituals, whether it is likely to be welcoming, and how confident others in the group are in communicating or being around a person with an intellectual disability. In terms of activities, inquiries need to be made. For example, are activities shared with other members, is there a common purpose, how might these be broken down into discrete tasks to facilitate engagement, what support might the person need to participate and who might provide this? This stage often requires negotiation with leaders of groups to gain entry and to assuage the reluctance that often comes with uncertainty and unfamiliarity with people with intellectual disabilities. The introductory period might involve staff providing some training or orientation to a group leader or members about the person's support needs. For example, members of a senior citizens group could be invited to be trained to mentor a new member with intellectual disability to ensure the new member knows the procedures for checking in, that someone says hello to them when they arrive and invites them to join one of the activities. Support from other members as natural supporters is much more likely to foster friendly social interaction than if

Table 4.1 Examples of convivial encounters and strategies to create them (adapted from Bigby & Anderson, 2021)

Identifying an opportunity for an individual and negotiating with a public institution or commercial enterprise
A young woman volunteers weekly in a local school replacing books on the shelves in the library. After a few weeks she is known by name by the teachers and many of the children in the school, who drop into the library to say hi to her.
Establishing a community service to a public institution and breaking down of process into discrete activities for a small group of people
A small group of people prepare fruit that has been discarded by a retailer and distribute it to each class in a school once a week. They cut up the fruit in the school kitchen and are welcomed by name by staff and pupils when they bring it to classrooms for the afternoon break.
Establishing a social enterprise and breaking down processes into discrete activities for a small group or individual
A young man regularly goes to collect jars purchased from a wholesaler to be filled with produce and sold in the organization's shop. He travels with a support worker and is recognized by the staff member at the wholesalers who is responsible for the order who asks him about his week and chats about work.
Identifying an opportunity for a group volunteer activity and negotiating with a commercial or public provider
Two people regularly volunteer with a local organization to deliver meals on wheels for older people. They take it in turns to get out of the van and bring meals to recipients' doors who recognize and thank them.
Identifying an opportunity for paid activity and negotiating with a commercial enterprise
Two people have a regular round delivering advertising material to letterboxes. They are recognized and greeted by people in the local area who are home during the day.
Identifying a suitable public facility or commercial place for an individual's preferred activity
One young woman goes swimming weekly in the local pool with a support worker. She has become friendly with an older man who goes at the same time each week and she often holds his hand and walks up and down the pool side with him.
Identifying an existing group for a preferred activity in a public facility, negotiating with facility staff
Two women go to a weekly water aerobics class at a local swimming pool, and over time gradually become more confident to attend without support from staff. After a while, they are recognized by people who sell tickets and greeted by other members of the class.
Creating a regular group or one-off activity for people with disabilities that is open to community members and people with intellectual disabilities in disability-specific, other specialist or mainstream spaces
A group of people who have been growing tomatoes invite community members to come to a chutney making day at the organization's shop. Some community members greet the people they recognize from the farm produce shop where they sell tomatoes once a week.

a person is accompanied by a support worker unfamiliar with the group and its culture. Training natural supporters was referred to as *Active Mentoring* in one program, as it drew on skills derived from Active Support and trained natural supporters in identifying moments of potential for engagement of the person, offering and respecting a person's choices and providing the right type and amount of assistance to ensure their successful completion of tasks.

Regularity is important in this type of program to help ensure the person gains confidence or skills in participating and becomes recognised and known by others. Once a person is included and comfortable attending regularly, program staff may only need to monitor how things are going and be ready to step in if something changes such as their mentor leaving, a class going into recess or an activity being rescheduled.

Programs that support convivial encounters can include people with higher support needs who will also require support to travel to and from a place. Program staff may also need to liaise with accommodation staff or families to ensure the activity is built into a person's regular routines. Further descriptions of programs that support convivial encounters are found in Bigby and Anderson (2021), (Craig & Bigby, 2015) and Stancliffe et al. (2013).

Emphasising a Sense of Identity and Belonging

Participating in some types of activities that happen in particular places creates new identities for people such as artists, craftspeople, singers or athletes and opens up membership of groups to which a person develops a sense of belonging. Belonging to a group creates opportunities for social interactions with peers as well as people without disability who have similar interests. If a program emphasises identity and belonging then strategies will focus on finding places where a person can further develop their talents, identity or share common interests with others. For example, in the earlier excerpts gaining an identity as an artist gave Elizabeth and John a sense of belonging and brought them into contact with other artists at exhibitions or events.

Programs to Support Identity and Belonging

These types of programs aim to create a sense of identity or belonging to a specific group or community of interest which in turn facilitates not only convivial encounters with immediate members of the group but with others beyond it who share a common identity or interest. Identities may be based on a person's creativity or talents (such as art, drama, singing or sport), or their status (for example as a self-advocate or peer). For instance, being a member of a football league for people with intellectual disabilities develops skills, brings people into touch with a regular group of peers and coaches interested in football and provides opportunities to be part of exhibition matches at bigger football events. Being a member of a self-advocacy group brings a person into touch regularly with other members and may provide opportunities to be part of other groups, such as advisory boards or delegations, to participate in conferences or to conduct training programs where a person might meet others with similar interests who belong to the wider community of people interested in disability rights.

Fostering a common sense of identity is the focus of programs that aim to further belonging. Some of the work of staff in these types of programs is organisational. For example, a program that supports people to participate in a drama group will need to manage the group's rehearsals and schedule performances. Some programs may need staff to have specialist skills in teaching, coaching or supporting the core activity. For example, an arts project employs artists as staff who use a technique called the 'hand in glove approach' to support the artist participants with intellectual disabilities. There may also be a process of recruiting participants to ensure they are a good fit for the program and understand what it offers as well as planning with them around their involvement and commitment.

Programs based on belonging or identity may only include people with intellectual disabilities as participants, such as Arts Project (Anderson & Bigby, 2021) or may include people with and without intellectual disability such as Tutti Arts described by Darragh et al. (2016). However, they always include activities that bring participants into contact with people without intellectual disabilities through, for example, exhibitions, performances or other types of events.

Practice Framework for Community Participation Programs

Despite the diversity of community participation, many have similar principles, processes and require staff to have a common set of skills, which can be brought together into a practice framework. This serves as a skeleton, setting out what must be considered when thinking about a program rather than a set of procedures or instructions. The framework proposed here includes principles that should inform all aspects of programs, processes that need to be incorporated into them and the skills that are necessary for successful implementation. This type of practice framework is useful for organisational leaders or managers to reflect on the design of new programs or those already on offer and the skills of the staff they employ; for support workers in understanding the processes they should undertake and the skills they need; and for people with intellectual disabilities and their families in thinking about choice and the quality of programs or in designing their own program. A framework may also be useful to regulators and funders in identifying components that comprise effective programs. The following sections describe the principles, processes and skills and knowledge central to a practice framework for community participation programs.

Principles

- *Reflecting individual preferences and support needs.* There is no ideal form of community participation. Programs support individuals to make choices about the places and activities and the people they prefer to interact with. Support is tailored to individual needs and the context in which a person lives.
- *Acknowledging the importance of engagement.* Programs support individuals to be engaged in activities and social interactions rather than simply to be present in community places.
- *Recognising the need for frontstage and backstage support.* Work behind the scenes (backstage)—planning, exploring possibilities, creating opportunities, negotiating, recruiting or preparing natural supporters or volunteers and monitoring—which precedes moments of participation determines success and is as important as direct (frontstage) support.
- *Collaborating with natural supporters.* Inviting others in a community context to collaborate to support inclusion. Working with natural supporters to develop their skills and confidence to support a person's participation can be more effective than relying on paid supporters, increases opportunities for social interaction and inclusion in

a group's culture, and may be more sustainable and reduce reliance on paid support over time.

- *Working in teams and being reflective.* Design and implementation of programs requires a mix of staff skills and relies on teamwork and reflective supervision to improve quality and develop staff skills.

Processes

- *Knowing the person and planning.* Person-centred planning with the person (and with their consent others who know them well) is undertaken for staff to get to know the person and establish their goals and preferences. Part of the planning process should include risk assessment and enablement strategies.
- *Exploring possibilities.* Options aligned with individual preferences and characteristics are explored. This might involve scanning communities of interest, identifying potential groups or places and analysing their culture or other characteristics, recruiting volunteers or even creating new groups or activities. It is important to understanding that regularity of participation and continuity of other participants are facilitators of engagement and social interactions.
- *Negotiating.* Matching a person to a group, negotiating their entry with leaders, sharing information if appropriate with leaders and other participants and offering training and support to natural supporters to enable inclusion. It may be necessary to build the activity into the person's schedule and coordinate with others involved in their support.
- *Supporting and maintaining.* Supporting the person to attend, and participate in the moment if necessary, monitoring their engagement over time and providing additional support if needed as the context or personal circumstances change.

Skills and Knowledge

- *Person-centred planning* skills including communication, listening, mapping networks and supporting decision-making.
- *Community development* skills and knowledge for backstage work include understanding different types of communities and their assets, networking, analysing and negotiating.

- *Micro support skills* for front stage work include evidence informed person-centred practices such as Active Support (see Chap. 7), Enabling Risk (Bigby et al. 2018, b) and Supported Decision Making (see Chap. 11).

Maximising Benefits of Community Participation Programs

Individualised funding, like that available through the NDIS, means that people with disabilities are likely to lead more varied lives than in the past when they might have attended a day program five days a week. The chances are they participate in a range of community activities, perhaps supported by several different programs. A challenge however, particularly in working with people with more severe intellectual disability, is *coordinating* aspects of a person's life and their various support providers. Coordination is important to avoid participation being disrupted by failures to respect the significance of being on time for participating in classes or groups, to support travel to places or preparedness to go out and to avoid conflicting demands on a person's time. Further, maintenance of a routine can be important for some people. As well as coordination to maximise regular participation, a further challenge is joining up fragmented insights about a person and sharing new knowledge about their preferences, interests or social connections derived from observing their experiences. This knowledge can be used by others to inform their support or contribute to future goals and planning. For example, if support workers in a group home know a person has a growing friendship with someone at a community class they might facilitate further social contact, or shared activities out of class hours with that person.

The individualised programs of the type described in this chapter help in furthering possibilities of interaction between people with and without disabilities and allaying stereotypical attitudes and uncertainty about including people with disabilities in everyday activities or places. In parallel, more systemic approaches to change are necessary to remove structural obstacles to community participation. There are dangers, however, that community-wide systemic change initiatives tackle highly visible obstacles such as physical or sensory access and neglect those that are less visible and more relevant to people with intellectual disabilities. These include, for example, issues of communication access where staff are unskilled in adjusting their modes of communication or where signage and information relies on people having literacy skills. Other examples of structural obstacles include:

- failures to recognise or adjust the pace or nature of classes or activities offered by community centres;
- unreliability or inaccessibility of public transport systems;
- a limited supply of accessible taxis; and
- poor designs of digital information, such as automated ticketing and phone enquiry systems that require complex problem-solving and literacy skills and do not have the option of talking to a person to assist with the process.

Despite the best intentions about accessibility, public facilities seldom adjust their practice sufficiently to enable participation of people with intellectual disabilities without support. Some research is also beginning to suggest that individualised funding may hold an inherent danger that, rather than developing their own expertise or bearing the costs of adjustment, mainstream programs or public facilities rely on individualised support to facilitate participation by people with intellectual disabilities (Wiesel et al., 2022). It takes skills and experience to apply a social model lens and identify the structural obstacles that particularly affect this group or recognise they can be remedied by systems change rather than just more individual support. Staff skilled in community participation programs are well placed to collaborate with other services and systems to identify the need for systemic changes and to remove obstacles through staff training, changing practices or adjusting infrastructure. Indeed, as well as individualised support, the role of such programs may extend to broader initiatives to develop greater accessibility of public infrastructure for people with intellectual disabilities and advocacy for systemic change.

Take Home Messages

- Support for community participation must be tailored to each individual and their interests.
- Community participation takes many different forms as does provision of support for participation, so it is important to be clear about what is expected to be achieved for the individuals you support.

- Engagement, including social interactions, are the hallmarks of community participation; simply being in a place or in a group are not the same as participating.
- Quality individualised support is likely to be delivered through well-designed programs and by skilled workers accountable to practice leaders.
- Behind the scenes or backstage work is important and may mean direct support in the moment from a paid worker becomes unnecessary or can be provided by other community members.

References

AIHW. (2022). *People with disability in Australia 2022*. Australian Government.

Amado, A. N. (2014). Building relationships between adults with intellectual disabilities and community members: Strategies, art, and policy. *Research and Practice in Intellectual and Developmental Disabilities, 1*(2), 111–122.

Anderson, S., & Bigby, C. (2021). Community participation as identity and belonging: A case study of arts project Australia. "I am an artist". *Research and Practice in Intellectual and Developmental Disabilities, 8*(1), 1–14.

Bigby, C. (2005). Comparative program options for aging people with intellectual disabilities. *Journal of Policy and Practice in Intellectual Disabilities, 2*(2), 75–85.

Bigby, C., & Anderson, S. (2021). Creating opportunities for convivial encounters for people with intellectual disabilities: "It looks like an accident". *Journal of Intellectual and Developmental Disability, 46*(1), 45–57.

Bigby, C., Anderson, S., & Cameron, N. (2018a). *Full report: Designing effective support for community participation for people with intellectual disabilities.* Report for Disability Research and Data Working Group.

Bigby, C., Clement, T., Mansell, J., & Beadle-Brown, J. (2009). 'It's pretty hard with our ones, they can't talk, the more able bodied can participate': Staff attitudes about the applicability of disability policies to people with severe and profound intellectual disabilities. *Journal of Intellectual Disability Research, 53*(4), 363–376.

Bigby, C., Douglas, J. M., & Vassallo, S. (2018b). *Enabling risk: Putting positives first. An online learning resource for disability support workers.* https://www.enablingriskresource.com.au

Bigby, C., & Wiesel, I. (2019). Using the concept of encounter to further the social inclusion of people with intellectual disabilities: What has been learned? *Research and Practice in Intellectual and Developmental Disabilities, 6*(1), 39–51.

Clement, T., & Bigby, C. (2010). *Group homes for people with intellectual disabilities: Encouraging inclusion and participation.* Jessica Kingsley Publishers.

Commonwealth of Australia. (2021). Australia's Disability Strategy 2021–2031.

Craig, D., & Bigby, C. (2015). "She's been involved in everything as far as I can see": Supporting the active participation of people with intellectual disability in community groups. *Journal of Intellectual and Developmental Disability, 40*(1), 12–25.

Darragh, J. A., Ellison, C. J., Rillotta, F., Bellon, M., & Crocker, R. (2016). Exploring the impact of an arts-based, day options program for young adults with intellectual disabilities. *Research and Practice in Intellectual and Developmental Disabilities, 3*(1), 22–31.

Fyffe, C., & Raskin, L. (2015). Design and implementation of a leisure buddy program. *Research and Practice in Intellectual and Developmental Disabilities, 2*(1), 83–91.

National Disability Insurance Scheme Act 2013 (NDIS), (2013).

NDIA. (2022). NDIS quarterly report to disability ministers, 2021–2022 fourth quarter, appendix A.

Stancliffe, R. J., Wilson, N. J., Gambin, N., Bigby, C., & Balandin, S. (2013). *Transition to retirement: A guide to inclusive practice*. Sydney University Press.

Verdonschot, M. M., De Witte, L. P., Reichrath, E., Buntinx, W. H., & Curfs, L. M. (2009). Community participation of people with an intellectual disability: A review of empirical findings. *Journal of Intellectual Disability Research, 53*(4), 303–318.

Wiesel, I., Bigby, C., van Holstein, E., & Gleeson, B. (2022). Three modes of inclusion of people with intellectual disability in mainstream services: Mainstreaming, differentiation and individualisation. *Disability and Society*, 1–22. https://doi.org/10.1080/09687599.2022.2060803

CHAPTER 5

The Importance of Economic Participation for Quality of Life

Vivienne C. Riches

Most societies place a high value on work and on all their citizens being gainfully employed, including people with disabilities. This is reflected in international conventions and national laws and policies of those Western countries that promote the employment of people with disabilities and protect them from discrimination. For example, the United Nations Convention on the Rights of People with Disabilities (CRPD) recognises that employment is a fundamental right of citizenship. Article 27 of the CRPD recognises:

> the right of persons with disabilities to work on an equal basis with others; this includes the opportunity to gain a living by work freely chosen or accepted in a labour market and work environment that is open, inclusive and accessible to persons with disabilities. (United Nations, 2006)

As a means of enacting this right, the CRPD prohibits all forms of employment discrimination, promotes access to vocational training and

V. C. Riches (✉)
Centre for Disability Studies (CDS), University of Sydney,
Camperdown, NSW, Australia
e-mail: vivienne.riches@sydney.edu.au

C. Bigby, A. Hough (eds.), *Disability Practice*,
https://doi.org/10.1007/978-981-99-6143-6_5

employment, and advocates for the use of strategies such as reasonable adjustments in workplaces (United Nations, 2006). Australia has a long history of policy and programmes promoting employment for people with disabilities; these are supported by measures to stop employers from discriminating against people with disabilities. For example, Australia's disability service system, the National Disability Insurance Scheme (NDIS), identified employment as a key expected outcome for people with disabilities eligible for the scheme (NDIS, 2020). Further, Australia's National Disability Employment Strategy (2021–2031) sets out a ten-year commitment to supporting jobseekers with disability to gain long-term, meaningful employment and address challenges that limit careers and access to employment.

Societal Benefits to Employing People with Disabilities

Greater workforce participation is viewed by governments as a key driving factor for economic growth, and competitive community-based employment of people with intellectual disabilities has proven to be a cost-effective option for government and society. Providing people with significant intellectual disabilities with the right support to work appears to be a significantly less costly alternative than day activity programmes that cater for a similar population; additional benefits include a reduction in disability pension costs, with support costs stabilising over time (Callahan et al., 2011). There is also strong evidence that workers with disabilities make good, dependable employees, who are highly motivated and can perform as well or better than their non-disabled peers on measures such as productivity, safety, and attendance (Lindsay et al., 2018). Their presence has often positively impacted a company's profitability and enhanced workforce morale. Furthermore, people with disabilities are more likely to stay in a job, which is important to employers who well know the costs of turnover, such as lost productivity, and the expenses related to recruitment and training. Companies also benefit by developing inclusive work cultures and improving disability awareness (ACCI, 2014).

Individual Benefits for People with Disabilities

Paid work is important for a person's economic security—which means not only escaping poverty (Nye-Lengerman & Nord, 2016) but covering essential needs sustainably and with dignity. Consequently, people with disabilities value earning an income and the financial independence it brings (Nord et al., 2013). Employment also contributes to many non-economic benefits that affect quality of life. Work is associated with better physical and mental health and well-being; greater autonomy, and choice and control; increased social status and social inclusion with opportunities to socialise and make friends; and an increased sense of belonging (Lindsay et al., 2018). Many people with intellectual disabilities have also reported they value work because it contributes positively to their sense of identity and self-worth, satisfaction, and self-confidence allowing them to contribute their gifts and talents in meaningful ways. Others appreciate the fact that work provides a structure and regular routine for everyday life that distinguishes work time from non-work time. Family quality of life can also be positively affected (Foley et al., 2013).

Employment Disadvantage

Unemployment is associated with many negative effects including poverty, social exclusion, poorer quality of life, and health and social inequalities (Nye-Lengerman & Nord, 2016). People with disabilities have much lower rates of participation in the workforce than the general population. In 2022, 53.4 per cent of Australians with disabilities were in the labour force compared to 84.1 per cent of people without disabilities. Their unemployment rate was 10.3 per cent, more than double that of people without disabilities (4.6 per cent) (AIHW, 2022). The situation is even worse for those with intellectual disabilities. According to Australian NDIS employment outcomes data, only 29 per cent of people with intellectual disabilities over 25 years and under 65 years were in paid employment when they entered the NDIS (Wilson & Campain, 2020). These rates are well below those of other countries and have not improved significantly since 2010. Australia ranks 19th among the 32 countries in the Organisation for Economic Cooperation and Development (OECD) for employment rates for people with disabilities. It ranks 22nd on the gap in employment rates between people with and without disabilities and 26th on the unemployment gap between people with and without disabilities (OECD, 2022).

Substantial under-employment also exists with one in ten people with disabilities, and one in six with intellectual disabilities, under-employed (AIHW, 2022). This occurs when jobs are part time or casual and people work fewer hours than they desire, resulting in financial strain. Under-employment also includes job roles and work tasks that require less skill than the employee possesses and when there are poor prospects of promotion. Such jobs are highly vulnerable to job loss during times of economic downturn. Under-employment has a serious negative impact on mental and physical health with high levels of dissatisfaction resulting in "rust out"—a health condition similar to burn out—where the person feels undervalued, under-utilised, and under-challenged (for example Blustein et al., 2013).

Employment Barriers and Opportunities

It is clear that high rates of unemployment and under-employment are not due to the capability or motivation of most people with intellectual disabilities, but to a variety of obstacles and barriers. Negative attitudes towards hiring people with disabilities, discrimination in the workplace, and stereotyping are common barriers that can affect all stages of employment. Negative parental attitudes to inclusive employment due to fears around discrimination, bullying, and safety can result in overprotection and directing school leavers to more segregated employment environments or alternative day programmes. Physical and architectural barriers also exist such as inaccessible workplaces and/or transport. Various technological and communication barriers may remain, despite developments in assistive technology such as prosthetics, text to speech, voice control, screen readers and magnifiers, and braille output devices. Even when technology solutions exist, individuals, their families, and employers may lack knowledge and/or the resources to access these. Policies and practices can also limit opportunities or inadvertently have a negative impact. For example, persons receiving an income-tested disability pension and their families can fear loss of this income support if they gain employment, and especially loss of crucial benefits such as reduced health and transport costs, especially when jobs are low paying and insecure.

Economic structural changes can have a far-reaching impact on employment, especially for vulnerable populations. The decline of jobs in manufacturing and agriculture and the shift to jobs in the services sectors has meant many people with intellectual disabilities have lowly paid and insecure jobs with poor career prospects in the service industries. The global Covid-19 pandemic negatively impacted economic participation for people with intellectual disabilities, especially in these jobs. Technological advances such as increasing use of automation, robotics, technology, and artificial intelligence are further reducing the availability of many jobs previously available to people with disabilities.

Nevertheless, new opportunities that break traditional stereotypes about disability employment are also emerging. For example, the fashion industry is raising awareness of adaptive clothing and promoting representation of people with disabilities in advertising, while increasing numbers of people with disabilities are working in the arts, film, TV, and media, and engaging in boutique businesses. Assistive technology solutions continue to emerge that can assist people in undertaking jobs not previously possible. Furthermore, many workplaces now recognise the value of diversity and inclusion and are developing policies and practices that can change workplace culture and create more diverse, disability-inclusive worksites.

Key Terms and Types of Disability Employment Programmes

Employment Preparation and Training Programmes

A range of work experience, transition from school to work, and vocational education and training (VET) programmes are available that can help prepare people with disabilities to acquire necessary work skills and be "job ready". These focus on important "soft skills" such as work habits and attitudes, communication, social skills, teamwork, and time management, as well as "hard skills" that are industry-specific job skills including technical, computer, or marketing skills.

Open Employment Programmes

Many countries have a range of government-funded and not-for-profit open employment programmes, also known as Competitive Integrated Employment (CIE). These programmes aim to help people find jobs where they work alongside people without disabilities, are paid the same as other workers, and have the same conditions of employment including benefits and opportunities for career progression.

Programmes can vary widely in type, quality, and outcomes achieved. Programmes support individuals to find and secure a regular job in open employment. Some programmes also provide short-term on-the-job training, especially for people with intellectual disabilities, and several provide ongoing post-placement support. Sometimes customised jobs are created that allow changes to the regular job role, work hours, and/or location to better suit the skills and circumstances of a particular person while still meeting the needs of the employer. Other programmes may use a co-worker model to support a person on the job. ***Self-employment and micro businesses*** (employing one to four people) offer greater control and flexibility but may require additional assistance with administration and finances.

Supported Employment Programmes

Supported employment programmes also aim to find people employment but provide long-term help and may pay lower wages. Programmes vary in size and auspice, as well as type of business model. Competitive supported employment programmes may employ individuals in inclusive mainstream labour market jobs; other supported employment programmes involve people working in a group with other people with disabilities such as enclaves, work crews, and social enterprises in more segregated settings. Continuous or intermittent on-the-job support and supervision are provided as needed. Participants in these less inclusive supported employment programmes often receive income support, getting a small wage. Jobs often involve packaging, assembly, production, recycling, screen-printing, plant nursery positions, garden maintenance and landscaping, cleaning services, laundry services, and food services. For example, a mobile work crew attached to a day programme allows a small group of workers to find and carry out contract gardening work in the community.

Sheltered Employment

Most countries have closed, or are in the process of closing or transitioning, sheltered workshops to supported employment models, but some large workshops still exist. These provide the most segregated or protected settings and pay the lowest wages. All Australian sheltered workshops have transitioned to become Business Services, also called Australian Disability Enterprises (ADEs).

Quality Practices and Programmes

Quality practices, also called "evidence-based practices" or good practices, inform us about what is effective if the practices are implemented correctly and faithfully over time. Quality practices are judged effective according to the best available evidence from rigorous international and national research studies. Evidence is increasingly available to support practices which align with values that treat people with disabilities (and their families) with respect and dignity, such as inclusive employment practices. There is a growing evidence base about practices that work well and practices that do not work when supporting people with intellectual and other disabilities to prepare for work and/or to find and keep a job of their choice. There are still some practices where there remains insufficient evidence to support widespread implementation.

Place-Then-Train Model

An important finding that affects all programmes involved in preparing and training people with intellectual disabilities for open and supported employment is the use of a place-then-train model. Contrary to the typical train-then-place model, where vocational training occurs before a person seeks and secures a job, the place-then-train employment model emphasises learning on-the-job and on-the-job support. This model has proven more effective and delivers better job placement and retention outcomes for people with intellectual disabilities—who may learn better through practical, hands-on experience—than train-then-place systems. Importantly, there is an abundance of evidence that previous extensive job readiness pre-vocational and vocational training curricula, which required people with intellectual disabilities to master a range of skills before they could progress or graduate to employment, were ineffective and locked people out of employment because they were never considered "ready" (Lewis et al., 2011). Even when skills were learnt in one environment, typically a classroom, difficulty generalising or transferring those skills from the classroom to the workplace meant that teaching and learning had to be repeated in the workplace. The readiness concept therefore proved to be a "readiness trap" that failed to produce employment outcomes.

Quality Support Personnel and Technical Assistance

Different terms are used for staff who work with disability employment programmes, including disability employment specialists, consultants, job coaches, and training officers. There is evidence that employment specialists, regardless of the programme type, job title, and specific role performed, are critical to programme success and good outcomes for workers with disabilities (Kregel et al., 2020; Laragy et al., 2013). Quality staff are person centred and believe in the capability of the people they support and their potential to be successfully employed. Disability employment specialists understand participants' needs and goals and use strength-based approaches that recognise that each person has their own unique abilities, gifts, and competencies. They are competent in the overall process of working with both the jobseeker and the employer, possessing the knowledge and skills necessary for their roles. A positive, can-do attitude to problems when they arise is also important, especially as personal obstacles and employment barriers can present challenges from time to time. Problem solving is recognised as an essential ingredient of the job, and not a nuisance that is interfering with the job, since people who view problems as an intrusion often respond in unproductive ways. Effective support personnel don't invite problems, but they do view them realistically and seek positive and creative ways to obtain successful outcomes.

Consequently, support staff training, professional development, and technical assistance are critical. Various online courses can provide knowledge, skills training, resources, and credentialling in areas such as instructional technology and applied behaviour analysis. In-house tailored staff training, networking, conference opportunities, and consultancies are other options for support staff to further their expertise.

Disability employment providers can also play a role in countering common myths and misconceptions and challenge negative attitudes that are a barrier to employment for people with disabilities. They can share resources such as fact sheets and promote disability employment as they work with employers and the public. Examples include disability awareness training programmes for employers and co-workers to improve their confidence in employing and working with a person with disability and developing disability-inclusive workplaces. They can provide assistance to employers to think creatively about ways jobs are structured and advise on and facilitate workplace modifications in the event these are needed (ACCI, 2014).

Quality Practices in Employment Preparation and Training Programmes

Transition Programmes

Transition programmes provide transition planning and vocational preparation for students in their final years of school and up to two years post-school to help students with disabilities refine their vocational interests and goals. These programmes assist students to develop realistic employment pathways and career goals and further develop their vocational skills. Transition from school to work programmes are often run in specialist schools for students with intellectual disabilities and in some mainstream education settings. Some post-school transition programmes are also available, such as Project Search, which is available in a number of countries, and the Australian School Leaver Employment Supports (SLES) programme, funded by the NDIS.

Quality transition-to-work programmes assist students and families to participate meaningfully in the transition planning process and support students to develop their own vocational goals and portfolios important for job applications. They will also teach relevant work habits and model attitudes to support successful employment, as well as support self-determination and assist with important functional life skills such as travel and money skills. There is some empirical evidence that school-based transition practices effectively raise expectations about succeeding in open employment and contribute to successful employment outcomes, especially for students with intellectual disabilities (Kregel et al., 2020).

Specific transition-to-employment practices associated with good outcomes for both school-based and post-school transition programmes are systematic and structured. They have the following characteristics:

- individualised, student-centred transition planning, where students choose their work and life goals;
- students' goals are used to guide the study programme in academic and hard and soft job skills, including, for example, improving social and communication skills, money handling, time management, and travel skills;
- there is family involvement in transition planning;

- substantial amounts of vocational training and work experience are delivered in real community worksites that match individual vocational strengths, preferences, interests and needs;
- job coaching or training in job tasks and soft skills such as social interaction with supervisors and co-workers is provided; and
- staff competencies support both the student and the employer.

There is no evidence that starting transition planning younger than 14 years of age improves employment outcomes (Kregel et al., 2020).

Vocational Education and Training

Vocational education and training (VET) courses offered by public and private providers of technical and further education can be suitable for some people with disabilities. VET courses provide the necessary certification and qualifications that are important for a job-focused pathway to a career and later career progression. Most courses are classroom based but can also provide first-hand experience in the workplace through an apprenticeship or traineeship. Disability consultants are sometimes available to support students with intellectual disabilities to undertake mainstream or special courses, and some disability employment providers can support individuals to obtain and complete apprenticeships or traineeships.

Outcome data about Australia's Nationally Accredited VET courses from Certificate Level 1 through to University Diploma level reveal that people with intellectual disabilities have very poor entry rates, course completion rates, and subsequent employment outcomes (NCVER, 2018). Nevertheless, there is evidence that completing a VET qualification increases the chances of employment and improves the chances of continuous job tenure two to three years after completion (Cavanagh et al., 2019).

Some people with intellectual disabilities can undertake mainstream courses successfully, while special courses for people with disabilities are sometimes available. Formal and informal supports are the most important factors facilitating course completion, and some programmes have consultants who can deliver disability-specific support to students. Learners with intellectual disability may struggle with classroom learning, and teachers require the knowledge and skills to recognise and respect differences in student needs and to adapt tasks and environments to support individual students. Inclusive curriculum design and practices are also required (Fossey et al., 2015).

University Options for People with Disabilities

Academically eligible students with disabilities can enrol in regular university courses. Many universities now have a disability inclusion action plan and disability consultants to assist with student learning, fair assessments, and reasonable adjustments. Students must disclose they have a disability to access supports.

Some countries offer specialised programmes of study for students with intellectual disabilities in segregated programmes on college campuses. An increasingly common type of programme in parts of Australia, Canada, some countries in Europe, and the USA supports students with intellectual disabilities to access an integrated tertiary education through colleges and universities. Although they may be academically ineligible to enrol in most regular programmes of study, students are admitted to tertiary institutions and given formal auditing status. This means they can audit units of study of their choice; participate as members of the class; and engage in the social, cultural, and sporting life of the college or university (O'Brien et al., 2019). Students are supported by a non-disabled peer, and a support facilitator navigates and buoys inclusion and assists academic staff in various ways. Some programmes provide specialised credentials, usually at the certificate level, that are not university accredited. Others conduct presentation events and award certificates of attendance or completion. Participants in these programmes may more confidently access regular pathways available for gaining a job following further education, including family and friend networks, recruitment agencies, work experience and mentorship programmes, or support from disability employment service providers.

Some programmes may also offer transition from university to employment and career support. One example is a "uni2beyond" initiative that partners with businesses and uses internship placements that enable interns to further explore career interests and advance their work-related skills and productivity. Person-centred career planning and on-the-job support are provided to the intern, while the host employer provides mentorship. Partner organisations also build their capacity through staff disability awareness training and the experience of participating in the programme (Riches et al., 2019).

Although general employment outcomes for tertiary students with disabilities fall well short of those achieved by graduates without disabilities, there is increasing evidence that individuals with and without disabilities who participate in university and college courses—even without obtaining a qualification—have superior employment outcomes, including a greater likelihood to gain employment and, additionally, earn a higher income compared to peers without tertiary education or experience (Marcotte et al., 2005). This includes students with intellectual disability and is especially the case when tertiary study was associated with collaborative support arrangements and programmes to transition from college or university to employment and a career.

Quality Practices for Open Employment

There is good evidence that open employment programmes that use the place-then-train model and a combination of four key practices achieve noticeably better outcomes when compared with alternative traditional job placement programmes and supported employment service types for people with intellectual disabilities (Kregel et al., 2020). Those outcomes include significantly higher employment rates, greater hourly earnings at or above minimum wage, and greater job retention over time. The four key practices required for successful job placement and retention are:

- personalised client assessment;
- individualised job development and placement;
- intensive training and support at the job site; and
- ongoing support throughout the course of the individual's employment.

Not one of these practices alone appears sufficient although it is possible that the prominence or weight of each of the four practices may vary between individuals. This is illustrated in the following discussion of the four practices and examples of their implementation.

Personalised Client Assessment

An effective assessment process provides the basis for an employment professional to help individuals become confident in their ability to succeed in employment, to refine their employment preferences, and to identify with the employment specialist the training and support necessary for success. A good assessment is both individualised and person centred and addresses specific job skills, work habits and attitudes, self-determination skills, and social and interpersonal relationships. The discovery model is one method designed to link the person's journey of discovery of their own interests, ambition, and potential, to the processes of job creation and ongoing supports. Assessment activities best occur in local job sites and other community settings based on the individual's employment goals, skills, strengths, and support needs.

The following case examples use pseudonyms and are based on research findings involving participants who were interviewed and observed on site.

Case Example

Richard's school referred him to a disability employment provider as he was keen to get a job and earn money. Together with his consultant, Gary, he explored his job interests, goals, and abilities. They identified interests in watching DVDs, going to the movies, and greeting and interacting with people. Richard's first goal was to work in a cinema, because he could meet people, watch lots of movies and earn money. However, when Gary helped him understand the conditions involved working nights and weekend shifts on a regular basis, he changed his mind as he preferred a day job and did not want to give up playing bowls on Saturdays with friends.

Richard and Gary then considered other interests and abilities with cooking and cleaning and a work experience food prep team member position was found at a local McDonalds. Richard learnt the job tasks and how to travel there on public transport. However he didn't like the job as he had to work long hours standing in the kitchen, and he became angry when everyone was bossing him around, "telling him what to do". These experiences were treated as learning and discovery opportunities, that helped Richard refine his work goals.

Individualised Job Development and Placement

This component involves strategies for developing and implementing an individualised job search plan based on the participant's assessment results, as well as job matching followed by job placement. Job matching involves evaluating job vacancies to check that the job duties, conditions, and production demands suit the individual or analysing jobs to determine their relevance to the strengths, interests, preferences, and needs of the individual.

Job analysis is a detailed and systematic process of breaking down work performed in an individual job into several separate tasks and duties. A good job analysis can identify opportunities for customising a position using strategies such as job creation, job carving (analysing tasks in a job role and swapping an element of the job duties to make the most of the person's skills), or job restructuring to suit the employer's needs as well as the skills and needs of the jobseeker. Information for the job analysis can be obtained by direct observation, working in the position to gain first-hand experience, and interviewing supervisors and co-workers and/or people who have done the job.

Effective job placements use information gained from both the job search and job matching strategies to ensure the job placement is a good match between the individual's skills, preferences, and choices and a standard or customised job. The detailed analysis of the position can also be presented to management to assist with their decision to offer employment. When arranging a placement for the jobseeker, it is important the employment specialist develops a positive relationship with the employer. This facilitates problem solving both during and after placement.

Case Example

Gary next found a local supermarket advertising a trolley collector position. The job analysis identified this did not require formal qualifications and would involve cleaning tasks in the store and collecting trolleys inside and from the outside carpark, no matter what the weather. Richard thought this could suit him as he liked being able to move around the workplace rather being in one place and working inside and outside. Collecting trolleys also meant only one supervisor would tell him what to do. Gary contacted the employer and negotiated a trial job working shifts from Monday to Friday.

Good practice when negotiating a placement involves the consultant presenting the business case for hiring workers with intellectual disabilities and the specific strengths of the participant. Based on the job analysis, participant support needs are shared and negotiated with the employer, including any job accommodations required, teaching and learning supports necessary, and how these could be delivered. For example, if job duties include handling money but this is not an option for the jobseeker, negotiation can occur to customise the job description by having this task reassigned to another position and replaced by tasks more suited to the participant's skills and abilities. Even when the employer may have their own training system, they may welcome the addition of skilled support from the employment specialist on the condition it is not intrusive to the workplace. Placement is followed by the implementation of personalised supports that will ultimately foster independence.

Intensive Training and Support at the Job Site

Quality job site instruction is based on principles of learning theory and applied behaviour analysis. Training and support are provided to ensure that all work tasks are completed at or above required standards and to the satisfaction of the employer and that social inclusion is promoted. Instructional strategies are matched to the person's unique support needs and typically include use of goal setting, step-by-step instruction using task analyses and/or checklists, graded levels of support with fading assistance to encourage greater independence, error correction procedures, and reinforcement strategies. Other effective vocational training techniques include video modelling of job tasks and/or social skills that allow the person to see how to perform steps correctly and in the right order; viewing own work performance by video feedback and discussing positive and negative aspects with the consultant; using audio prompts provided discreetly during job training and/or checklists using words, pictures, or graphics to schedule the sequence and timing of tasks and job duties; self-management strategies for emotional regulation; and utilising a wearable watch alarm for time management.

Ongoing Support Throughout the Course of the Individual's Employment

In programmes where ongoing support is provided, the needs of both the participant and the employer are addressed for as long as the person remains employed. Assistance is based on needs and requests from either party and can fluctuate over time in frequency and intensity. Coping with changes in management or supervisory arrangements or assigned tasks may require support or training. Good on-the-job support is discreet and aims to minimise disruption to workflow or relationships with work colleagues, supervisors, or the employer. Additional support may be provided off site.

Case Example
The employer was happy for Gary to train Richard to learn the cues for when to collect the trollies, accept instructions, schedule cleaning tasks, and assess productivity. The employer had its own training program to teach cleaning and chemical use. Richard quickly learnt the various tasks involved including using the cleaning equipment. By the end of one month Gary assessed Richard was performing all job tasks and routines competently. The employer was very happy with his performance and felt he was an asset to the store. Richard was enjoying the job, especially being able to say hello to customers when collecting and returning trolleys. Gary initially reduced his visits to checking in with Richard on site after each shift and then moved to weekly check-ins. After three months the employer was satisfied with Richard's work and his ability to relate well to the customers, many of whom commented how helpful he was, and he was offered a permanent position. Richard and the employer had Gary's mobile so either could contact him if any problems arose. Last reports were that Richard has won several "employee of the month" awards and is saving money for a special holiday.

Quality Practices and Supported Employment

Many of the good practices described above are common to both open and supported employment. Additionally, there is good evidence that the Individual Placement and Support (IPS) model of competitive supported employment is effective for people with intellectual disabilities and severe mental illness (Bond et al., 2000). Key practices include zero exclusion (the only requirement is motivation to work), attention to consumer choice and preferences, rapid job search, integrated mental health and vocational services for people with severe mental illness, appropriate levels of individualised support, and counselling about how employment may impact government benefits and income support. Benefits counselling is usually necessary because participants can fear losing income support or other benefits if employed.

The social enterprise model aims to provide people with intellectual disabilities dignity and respect, a socially valued role in the community, a career rather than just a job, and the capacity to deliver higher wages (Meltzer et al., 2018; Smith et al., 2018). Good practices in social enterprises focus on building skills to help participants enter the mainstream job market. This model can provide encouragement, understanding, and good connections with the community, as well as structured training, work experience, or work placement with a focus on paid employment.

Less inclusive and more protected settings can be preferred by some individuals and their families due to fear of discrimination and bullying. They can also offer easier access to work, and greater job stability and job security. However, relatively few workers have moved from sheltered workshops to open employment, so it should not necessarily be viewed as a stepping stone to open employment.

Linking with Related Service Systems

Many other areas can impact a person's ability to gain and maintain employment. Consequently, people with disabilities, their families, and staff often need information on a range of related services. This includes understanding human rights and responsibilities, especially the right to be respected, to be safe, and to be treated fairly in the workplace and community. It may also include engaging with the case for and against disability disclosure and what to do about discrimination, bullying, or grievances. Various advocacy groups, peak organisations, and specific disability organisations exist that can provide advocacy, support, and resources for the disability employment sector.

Good health and well-being, a stable place to live, accessible transport, social relationships, community connections, and lifestyle patterns are important interrelated areas that may need to be considered. Linkages to information and access to various resources or services run by government and non-government organisations may be required across a range of areas including housing, counselling, financial planning and management, health and medical services and benefits, and travel. Some countries provide financial supports to people with disabilities, such as a disability pension, health benefits, and travel concessions. Support programmes need to ensure individuals understand any benefit schemes available and also the potential disadvantage of reliance on such assistance at the expense of employment to avoid a "poverty trap" that keeps people economically disadvantaged.

Conclusion

Improving disability employment makes good business and economic sense to governments, employers, people with disabilities, and their families alike, yet the current employment picture for people with intellectual and other disabilities worldwide is equivocal. On the one hand, employment is widely recognised as a human right, and government policies and legislation strongly support full accessibility and inclusion on an equal basis with others. On the other hand, significant unemployment and under-employment rates prevail. Various barriers exist that continue to require attention, yet new and emerging employment possibilities are breaking traditional stereotypes and providing fresh perspectives that showcase peoples' strengths and abilities.

Importantly, there is a wealth of evidence that people with intellectual and other disabilities can gain successful outcomes in open and supported employment when tailored and quality practices are used. Quality practices need to be implemented faithfully by knowledgeable and skilled disability employment providers who work with both the individual with a disability and the employer to achieve desired outcomes. This leads to a better quality of life for the individual and the family, with fair wages for real work. Businesses also benefit by gaining motivated, reliable, and productive employees whose valued presence can improve productivity, increase satisfaction of both employers and employees, and enhance workplace culture.

Take-Home Messages

- Greater economic participation of people with disabilities is important for society, business, and individual quality of life.
- People with intellectual disabilities make good, dependable employees, who can perform as well or better than their non-disabled peers on measures such as productivity, safety, and attendance.
- Barriers contributing to high unemployment and under-employment need to be reduced and new opportunities created and further explored.

- Open employment leads to measurably better employment outcomes compared to other service approaches, but outcomes between providers still vary widely.
- Good support practices are strength based and tailored to meet individual interests, abilities, skills, and learning needs.
- Quality employment practices for people with intellectual disabilities involve a place-then-train model and a combination of components addressing assessment, job matching, on-the-job training, and assistance and ongoing support.

References

ACCI. (2014). *Employ outside the box: The business case for employing people with disability*. Australian Chamber of Commerce and Industry.

AIHW. (2022). People with disability in Australia 2022 [report]. *Australian Institute of Health and Welfare*. https://doi.org/10.25816/5ec5be4ced179

Blustein, D. L., Kozan, S., & Connors-Kellgren, A. (2013). Unemployment and underemployment: A narrative analysis about loss. *Journal of Vocational Behavior, 82*(3), 256–265. https://doi.org/10.1016/j.jvb.2013.02.005

Bond, G. R., Picone, J., Mauer, B., Fishbein, S., & Stout, R. (2000). The quality of supported employment implementation scale. *Journal of Vocational Rehabilitation, 14*(3), 201–212.

Callahan, M., Griffin, C., & Hammis, D. (2011). Twenty years of employment for persons with significant disabilities: A retrospective. *Journal of Vocational Rehabilitation, 35*(3), 163–172.

Cavanagh, J., Meacham, H., Cabrera, P. P., & Bartram, T. (2019). Vocational learning for workers with intellectual disability: Interventions at two case study sites. *Journal of vocational education & training, 71*(3), 350–367. https://doi.org/10.1080/13636820.2019.1578819

Foley, K. R., Jacoby, P., Girdler, S., Bourke, J., Pikora, T., Lennox, N., Einfeld, S., Llewellyn, G., Parmenter, T. R., & Leonard, H. (2013). Functioning and post-school transition outcomes for young people with down syndrome. *Child Care Health and Development, 39*(6), 789–800. https://doi.org/10.1111/cch.12019

Fossey, E., Chaffey, L., Venville, A., Ennals, P., Douglas, J., & Bigby, C. (2015). Supporting tertiary students with disabilities: Individualised and institution-level approaches in practice. Research report. NCVER.

Kregel, J., Wehman, P., Taylor, J., Avellone, L., Riches, V., Rodrigues, R., & Taylor, D. (2020). A comprehensive review of evidence-based employment practices for youth and adults with intellectual and other developmental disabilities. Rehabilitation Research and Training Center at Virginia Commonwealth University in Richmond, Virginia and Centre for Disability Studies, affiliated with the University of Sydney, Australia.

Laragy, C., Ramcharan, P., Fisher, K., McCraw, K., & Williams, R. (2013). *Making it work: A workforce guide for disability service providers.*

Lewis, G., Thoresen, S. H., & Cocks, E. (2011). Successful approaches to placing and supporting apprentices and trainees with disability in Australia. *Journal of Vocational Rehabilitation, 34*(3), 181–189.

Lindsay, S., Cagliostro, E., Albarico, M., Mortaji, N., & Karon, L. (2018). A systematic review of the benefits of hiring people with disabilities. *Journal of Occupational Rehabilitation, 28*(4), 634–655. https://doi.org/10.1007/s10926-018-9756-z

Marcotte, D. E., Bailey, T., Borkoski, C., & Kienzl, G. S. (2005). The returns of a community college education: Evidence from the National Education Longitudinal Survey. *Educational Evaluation and Policy Analysis, 27*(2), 157–175. https://doi.org/10.3102/01623737027002157

Meltzer, A., Kayess, R., & Bates, S. (2018). Perspectives of people with intellectual disability about open, sheltered and social enterprise employment: Implications for expanding employment choice through social enterprises. *Social Enterprise Journal, 14*(2), 225–244. https://doi.org/10.1108/SEJ-06-2017-0034

NCVER. (2018). Total VET students and courses 2017 [Report]. National Centre for Vocational Education Research. https://apo.org.au/node/184456

NDIS. (2020). *Employment outcomes for NDIS participants.*

Nord, D., Luecking, R., Mank, D., Kiernan, W., & Wray, C. (2013). The state of the science of employment and economic self-sufficiency for people with intellectual and developmental disabilities. *Intellectual and Developmental Disabilities, 51*(5), 376–384. https://doi.org/10.1352/1934-9556-51.5.376

Nye-Lengerman, K., & Nord, D. (2016). Changing the message: Employment as a means out of poverty. *Journal of Vocational Rehabilitation, 44*(3), 243–247.

O'Brien, P., Bonati, M. L., Gadow, F., & Slee, R. (2019). *People with intellectual disability experiencing university life: Theoretical underpinnings, evidence and lived experience*. Brill.

OECD. (2022). *Disability, work and inclusion*. Organisation for Economic Cooperation and Development. https://doi.org/10.1787/1eaa5e9c-en

Riches, V., Gadow, F., & MacDonald, J. (2019). Transition from university to employment. In P. O'Brien (Ed.), *People with intellectual disability experiencing university life : Theoretical underpinnings, evidence and lived experience* (pp. 255–266). Brill.

Smith, P., McVilly, K. R., McGillivray, J., & Chan, J. (2018). Developing open employment outcomes for people with an intellectual disability utilising a social Enterprise framework. *Journal of Vocational Rehabilitation, 48*(1), 59–77.

United Nations. (2006). *Convention on the Rights of Persons with Disabilities (CRPD)*. UN General Assembly.

Wilson, E., & Campain, R. (2020). *Fostering employment for people with intellectual disability: The evidence to date.* Centre for Social Impact, Swinburne University of Technology.

CHAPTER 6

Relationship-Based Practice with People with a Mild Intellectual Disability Who Have Been Socially Marginalised and Excluded

Kathy Ellem and Jemma Venables

This chapter focuses on a group of people who do not always identify as disability service users, yet nonetheless require support to enjoy a successful life in the community. This diverse group of people, hereafter referred to as people with a mild intellectual disability, may have been given a number of diagnostic labels, including foetal alcohol spectrum disorder, learning disability, autism spectrum disorder, traumatic brain injury, acquired brain injury, borderline intellectual functioning, or borderline intellectual disability. Many of this group also have co-occurring psychiatric conditions, including depression, anxiety disorders, psychosis, personality disorders, and addictive disorders (Ellem, 2019). In addition, this group often present with complex support needs related to adverse life experiences, such as homelessness, violence, involvement with child protection and criminal legal systems, and complex behaviours which can include harm to

K. Ellem (✉) • J. Venables
School of Nursing, Midwifery and Social Work, The University of Queensland, St Lucia, QLD, Australia
e-mail: k.ellem@uq.edu.au; jemma.venables@uq.edu.au

C. Bigby, A. Hough (eds.), *Disability Practice*,
https://doi.org/10.1007/978-981-99-6143-6_6

self or others and substance misuse (Dowse et al., 2019). This chapter draws on case studies from the authors' experiences as social work practitioners and service users, as well as findings from previous research. The examples are deidentified and adapted from these sources and do not represent any one individual.

A person with a mild intellectual disability can engage with multiple service sectors, including disability, health, education, criminal legal, drug and alcohol, mental health, and homelessness services. These interactions with service providers may be at a point of crisis—for example, a person seeking medical assistance at a hospital emergency department. The point of service contact can also be an involuntary client, such as someone who has been arrested by police for disorderly behaviour.

The diagnostic labels given to a person with a mild intellectual disability are usually only one part of a person's identity, and many may not identify with or embrace these labels at all. The following example illustrates this:

> Angela is a 22-year-old Aboriginal woman with a mild intellectual disability. Her child was removed from her care at birth and the records from the child protection office state that she is "mentally retarded". Angela equates this label with what she regards as unfair removal of her child. She prefers to see her disability as behavioural, given all the trouble she had at school. Her worker needs to arrange a psychological assessment for Angela if she is to apply for National Disability Insurance Scheme (NDIS) funding. This will involve talking through with Angela why the assessment is needed and what is involved, all the time honouring Angela's cultural identity, how she describes her needs, and the trauma she has experienced in losing her child.

In the example above, the diagnostic labels given to Angela are associated with the loss of a child and have no cultural relevance to Angela as an Aboriginal woman. This shows how labels can be regarded as stigmatising to the person and be associated with traumatic events where a person has been discriminated against or denied support from others.

A further complicating factor about diagnostics labels is that many people's disability may not be adequately assessed. Without proper assessment, many people with a mild intellectual disability miss out on formal supports and are deemed ineligible for disability support services such as the National Disability Insurance Scheme (NDIS). Even if a person is assessed by a professional, the complexity of their presentation may make it difficult to determine an accurate diagnosis. The professional may misattribute a person's symptoms to certain diagnoses and overlook other important indicators—a response often described as "diagnostic overshadowing". Interestingly, a person's disability may not be identified at all, as the person may present as competent and independent and mask what difficulties they experience (Wieland & Zitman, 2016). Regardless of these problems in disability identification, a person with a mild intellectual disability often needs some support with activities of daily living. This support can be in relation to adaptive behaviour—they may need help with practical life skills (e.g., cooking, cleaning, managing money), social skills (such as relating to others), and conceptual skills (e.g., communication and self-direction). A person may also experience challenges in executive functioning, the higher-order thinking processes involved in problem solving, reasoning, planning, memory, self-regulation, and learning from experiences.

Why Are Relationships Important to Good Quality of Life?

While it is important to understand how a person's disability may affect them at a functional level, it is also essential to understand the social and environmental context in which people live. The well-being of people with a mild intellectual disability is significantly influenced by their interactions with others around them, including their intimate social networks, and their relationship with services and systems. Quality of life can be measured in part by the nature of a person's interactions with their social world and by the degree to which a person feels that they belong and can actively participate in their community. Positive and supportive interactions with others can lead to increased community engagement, a stronger sense of self-worth, and increased resilience to face life challenges.

Many people with a mild intellectual disability occupy marginalised social positions within their communities, and therefore relationships with others can be quite poor. People with a mild intellectual disability can experience significant social disadvantage in relation to unemployment, poverty, poor educational experiences, substandard physical and mental health, and complex family histories. They may also experience higher rates of abuse, violence, and exploitation in relationships with others than the general population. They may have had involvement with the child protection system as a child and as a parent of a child in care, and they may have interacted with criminal legal systems as victims and alleged offenders (McManus et al., 2018). They may have experienced many dehumanising encounters with others and internalised the messages they receive, leading them to question their own value as human beings. Because of their life experiences, people with a mild intellectual disability can develop ineffective coping strategies to life, which can include impulsive problem behaviour, addictions, and acts of harm and violence to themselves and others.

What Are the Roles of Support Services in Relationship-Based Work?

Positive, life-affirming relationships are a precious resource for everyone, including people with a mild intellectual disability. Helpful relationships provide the context for a person to take control over their own life decisions, access support and information, and build their social connections and belonging (Ellem et al., 2013). Support services, both within the disability sector and within other sectors, can engage in relationship-based developmental work which focuses on these aims. This type of work is not limited by prescriptive interventions or "techniques" but focuses on the quality of relationship with people with an intellectual disability. This approach works at several levels:

- At the personal level, the focus is on improving interactions between support workers and the individuals they work with, as well as supporting and enhancing the individual's relationships with their family, friends, and community.
- At the organisational level, the culture of a service should support relationship-based developmental work, with resources and training directed to this end.
- At a service/systems level, relationship-based developmental work should occur between services and systems to ensure cross-agency collaboration and integrated service delivery.

Each of these levels are discussed in more detail below, with some suggestions for practice.

Relationship-Based Practice at the Personal Level

Working with Individuals

Poor life experiences can cause a person with a mild intellectual disability to withdraw from social interaction and relationships, and people may become hesitant to access support services. Feeling socially disconnected can make one feel unsafe and hyper-vigilant for social threats. There may be feelings of distrust towards support services if there has been a history of rejection, and a tendency to either avoid engagement in programmes (that is, the "flight" response) or be openly hostile to professional assistance (the "fight" response) (McConnell et al., 2016). The chaos a person experiences in their everyday life may place them in a perpetual state of crisis, and their personal energy to engage with professionals may be deeply compromised (Ellem et al., 2020).

Support workers' initial encounters with people with a mild intellectual disability must therefore be sensitive and careful, and considerable time must be taken to establish rapport, illustrated here with Rachel's interaction with Kim:

> Rachel is a 17-year-old young person with a mild intellectual disability and autism who has been referred to a disability service that supports young people with a history of child protection involvement. Kim, the worker from the service, wants to invite Rachel to a regular group where she can connect to other young people with similar experiences. Rachel is suspicious about Kim's motives, and sees her as another person from welfare telling her what to do, not to smoke, etc. Kim turns up to Rachel's school at the same time each week. At first it is just to say "hi" and to say she will drop in next week. Kim reads how Rachel is responding to her and reassures her that she doesn't have an issue with her smoking, as she knows Rachel understands it is bad for her health. Rachel sees that Kim is allowing her freedom to make her own choices and she is willing to give the group a go.

Rachel's story highlights that in the initial stages of the helping relationship, the worker may need to take a persistent but gentle approach to engaging with a person. This might involve meeting the person in an environment where they feel comfortable and the worker having a regular presence that is respectful and non-judgemental. It may involve the worker sharing, in a safe way, aspects of their own personal life they feel comfortable discussing. This helps overcome power inequalities in the relationship and to build connection and trust (Healy, 2018).

To truly be helpful, a worker needs to take time to learn about the core messages in a person's life. These core messages are what can drive a person to act in certain ways, which on the surface may seem contradictory to what the person really wants or needs (Ellem et al., 2013). For example, a person with a mild intellectual disability may experience a lot of powerlessness in their life and therefore feel the need to assert themselves with others. They may do so by saying "no" to things they actually want. Behaviours that others may find difficult or confronting can be regarded as a form of communication and are clues to a person's core messages. A skilled worker seeks to understand what the person is really communicating, taking note of any emotional issues underlying the behaviour. With this understanding, the worker can gently assist the person to find more pro-social means to attain what they need. As shown in Allan's story below, the core messages of the person therefore provide guidance as to the purpose of the helping relationship:

> Allan, a 27-year-old man with autism and a mild intellectual disability, has expressed to his worker that he would like to have a girlfriend. Jim, Allan's worker, finds out about a group which supports people with autism to learn about dating and friendship. When Jim asks Allan about it, he says "no". Jim thinks the "no" may be related to Allan not knowing what the group is about, and not feeling comfortable going to a new place. Jim decides to raise the opportunity again to Allan when he mentions about wanting a girlfriend, but this time he offers to take Allan there to ask the group leader some questions. He also offers to come along to the group with Allan until he feels comfortable attending alone.

The worker in relationship-based practice holds their commitment to the helping relationship and draws upon their own personal resources to do so. Such work requires a great deal of time, reflection, honesty, perseverance, observation, open-mindedness, and creativity (Collings et al., 2015). It also involves a realistic evaluation on the part of the worker that they play only one small part in the person's life and that it is the person themselves who has the resilience and skills to address the issues facing them (Caouette et al., 2018). The worker's role is often to question commonly held social beliefs about people with learning difficulties, which paint people as incapable and overly dependent on others. Instead, the worker facilitates sufficient time and space, experiences, and information for the person with an intellectual disability to chart their own course and live their life on their own terms.

Relationship-based practice takes advantage of naturally occurring situations to build connection with people, to help them to build knowledge, and to make decisions about their lives. The practical tasks that workers engage in with people with a mild intellectual disability, such as driving them to an appointment or helping a person go shopping, present multiple opportunities for connection. These everyday situations potentially connect a person to their local community and help them learn important life skills. They also provide a sense of safety for a person to open up about what is happening in their life and to discuss ways of problem-solving issues with the worker. These times can also be opportunities to share common interests and to give the person with a mild intellectual disability a reprieve from some of the intense issues they may be currently facing. As shown in Mitali's story below, what others may see as simple, menial tasks in disability support work thus become laden with purpose and meaning for the relationship-oriented support worker:

> Mitali has started providing support to Amy, a 30-year-old single mum with a mild intellectual disability. Amy's children are in the care of child protection services, but they are allowed to visit their mum and eventually Amy hopes to have her children stay with her overnight. For this to happen, Amy needs to learn how to better manage her pension money and ensure that she has enough food in the house. On one of her visits, Mitali drives Amy to get a food parcel from a local charity. While this does not appear to be getting to the core of the issue about where Amy's money is going, it is a critical opportunity for Mitali to connect with Amy. The car is a safe space for Amy to open up about things that are happening in her life, it can be a space where Mitali and Amy can listen and enjoy music together, and most importantly it is an opportunity for Mitali to understand what is important to Amy.

Relationship-based work also involves extending both the reach and range of relationships for a person with learning difficulties (Ellem et al., 2013). The work is often also with significant others in the person's life. It may involve building new understandings in existing family and friendship relationships, such as assisting in resolving conflict or facilitating reconnection. Sometimes this work can be extremely challenging. When a person with a mild intellectual disability is in an abusive or exploitative relationship with someone, it may involve the worker, with the person's consent, making their presence known to the abuser and shining a light on the behaviour. This approach is exampled by Andrew's story:

> Andrew is 31 years old, has a mild intellectual disability and lives in a unit in a public housing complex. Andrew tells his worker Sam that there is a new tenant downstairs in the public housing complex named Richard. Andrew said Richard gave him a lift to the automatic teller machine (ATM) the other day and asked Andrew for some money for smokes. Andrew gave him the money but felt a bit uncomfortable about it. Sam talks through with Andrew about how important it is to keep your money transactions private. Sam makes a note to visit Andrew at the complex and to say hello to Richard while she is there. She wants to get to know Richard more, to casually mention how nice it was of Allan to lend him money when he is only on a pension, and to let Richard know of her ongoing presence and support in Allan's life.

In such circumstances, the safety and well-being of the person with a mild intellectual disability is paramount, but it is often unrealistic to persuade the person to disassociate from the other person. Rather, it involves the worker suspending their own judgement of the situation. The worker has a role in seeking to accentuate the positives in the relationship while helping the person with a mild intellectual disability to establish some boundaries with the other person. If the relationship ends, it is hoped that this is a decision made by the person with a mild intellectual disability and not something imposed on them. When people are given the space to make their own decisions about relationships, they are more likely to learn how to keep themselves safe and to establish healthy boundaries with others.

Groupwork

Relationship-based practice at the personal level can also entail the facilitation of intentional groupings of people with an intellectual disability. Groupwork is an opportunity to collectively recognise and make the most of underutilised gifts in each group member (McMaster, 2016). Such groupwork has the most value when people with an intellectual disability have ownership over the group and can determine the purpose of gathering. Activities within a group setting will have different meanings to each individual group member. One person may benefit from learning practical skills in group activities, such as cooking and money management. Another person may use the space to practise social skills and build confidence to work collaboratively with others. Groupwork can also be a valuable opportunity for people to become familiar with other workers in the organisation, to mentor others in the group, to come together collectively around issues that are important to the group as a whole, and to engage in advocacy (Anderson & Bigby, 2017). Examples of successful groups have been highlighted by authors, such as self-advocacy groups (Ellem et al., 2022) and supported social groups (Wilson et al., 2017).

The coming together of people with difficult life histories can create an added complexity to groupwork. The role of group facilitators is therefore to create a safe space for all members of the group. This often involves individual support given to a person both prior to attending the group and in parallel to the group. Workers can assess a person's readiness and willingness to be involved and ensure the person does not have extenuating circumstances that prevent them from participating. Any agreements made collectively about how the group should operate should ensure that people with a mild intellectual disability have the time and space to express their ideas and comprehend what may be asked of them. The group space above all needs to be welcoming of all members and be flexible enough to allow people to join the group in their own time. Facilitators need to undertake proactive safety planning and devise exit strategies for people from the group environment if a person's comments or behaviours are triggering for others within the group. Group facilitators also need to ensure the ratio of workers to people with an intellectual disability is optimal so that the group is not dominated by the voices and priorities of paid staff, yet there is an opportunity for a person with a mild intellectual disability to seek one-on-one support away from the group should they need it.

All of the above examples of relationship-based practice require a significant investment on the part of service providers, in terms of time, funding, and commitment to quality practice. The next section discusses ways in which services can create a suitable environment for such work at the organisational level.

Relationship-Based Practice at the Organisational Level

Organisational policies and practices can support relationship-based practice with people with a mild intellectual disability. Decisions made and actions undertaken at the organisational level influence the types of supports offered and the overall outcomes for this group of people. As previously mentioned, many people with a mild intellectual disability are deemed ineligible for disability support services based on their disability diagnosis. They may also be actively excluded from programmes due to their complex support needs. Service providers may become "risk-averse" to clients with a history of complex behaviours and/or criminal legal system involvement. Managers of services may question the capacity and skill set of their staff to respond appropriately to behaviours that may challenge, and there may be concerns about ensuring the safety of staff and other service users. These pressures may be exacerbated by funding models, such as Australia's NDIS, which emphasises market-place competition and flexibility and autonomy within the disability support workforce. This has seen the emergence of business service models which are contractual in nature, rely on online platforms for the direct recruitment of disability support staff, and increase the casualisation of the disability services workforce. Within such contexts it becomes difficult to appoint, train, and supervise key workers with higher-level skills/qualifications who can work holistically with people with a mild intellectual disability.

Given these challenges, a key consideration in improving the lives of people with a mild intellectual disability involves improving their access to support. Service providers in all sectors need to develop proactive strategies to ensure they cater for this group of people. For services where people with a mild intellectual disability represent a small proportion of the clientele, such as housing services and health services, this may involve the development of service information in Easy English formats to assist a person to understand what supports are on offer and what the person's rights are in regard to the organisation. For services which position people with a mild intellectual disability as involuntary clients—for example, child protection and criminal legal services—improving access to support is likely to involve advocacy representation for the person, such as the inclusion of an independent third party who can safeguard the person's rights. Disability services can engage in outreach practices which involve actively reaching out to people with a mild intellectual disability in the everyday places they occupy in their communities rather than always relying on referrals from other service providers (Grymonprez et al., 2017).

The widening of eligibility criteria in disability service programmes and flexibility in assessment processes can greatly assist people with a mild intellectual disability to receive support. Eligibility should not only consider a person's diagnosis but also account for any challenges in the person's social circumstances. All service providers, regardless of the type of service, should seek to minimise bureaucratic processes for the service user, which may serve to alienate and confuse people with a mild intellectual disability.

The organisational space of all services needs to be a safe, welcoming environment for those it intends to support. It is beneficial if services are located close to public transportation and to other relevant services. By considering all these elements, the service user with an intellectual disability can establish relationships with staff members and a relationship with the place in which those staff members work.

The model of service delivery can also be influential in ensuring a stable and supportive response to people with a mild intellectual disability. A disability service provider can designate key workers for people within this group. From the perspective of the service user, a key worker can offer consistency and continuity in support and can become the point of contact when help is needed. The key worker can provide guidance to other support workers for the person and can assist the person in their communication and interaction within other service contexts and stakeholders. The service provider can support the worker to have frequent and regular contact with service users and not place unhelpful time limits on the duration of the helping relationship (Renehan et al., 2017). However, other workers should also be encouraged to connect with service users with a mild intellectual disability so that each person has a familiar face to contact in the event that the key worker is unavailable.

To truly embody the principles of relationship-based practice, it involves consideration and respect for all stakeholders. Organisations need to recognise the gifts and abilities of both with a mild intellectual disability and their workers if relationship-based practice is to prosper. A failure to commit to service users and staff to carry through relationship-based practice can lead to poor outcomes. For example, the recruitment and retention of skilled disability support workers is crucial yet challenging in a sector which is known for high levels of casualisation in the workforce and low levels of remuneration (Robinson et al., 2022). Staff need to work within a supportive organisational culture and context to truly help their service users. Similarly, organisations should value the voices and input from people with a mild intellectual disability and their families in their decision-making and governance. The input of service users into organisational decisions can help a service to keep its focus on improving the lives of people with an intellectual disability.

To sustain relationship-based practice, service providers need to actively build the knowledge base of both people with a mild intellectual disability and workers and provide appropriate training opportunities. Knowledge, for both workers and people with an intellectual disability, is derived from many sources and can include technical knowledge (such as learning how to keep a budget or run a meeting), story-telling (such as the sharing of practice examples or case studies), knowledge from lived experience (such as when giving people the opportunity to try something new), and knowledge from conscious reflection (such as critical reflection activities for workers). When the source of knowledge is considered in this way, opportunities for training and skill development can be diverse. The building of knowledge can be a collective event—for example, running a service provider forum related to overarching policy and practice initiatives in the disability sector—or it could be person-specific—such as behavioural support strategies related to individual service users or specific training development needs identified by a staff member in supervision. The sharing of knowledge can also involve peer-mentoring between staff members, and knowledge translation can be led by people with a mild intellectual disability.

Good supervision, a component of knowledge-building, is indispensable in relationship-based practice and can support a worker's emotional and professional growth (Rasmussen & Mishna, 2018). Supervision can take many forms, including critical reflection groups and activities with workers, informal peer supervision, incidental debriefing, and formal individual supervision. The key to such practices is to foster an organisational culture in which workers can take risks, safely discuss their mistakes, and learn from them. Supervision is also a forum in which managers can monitor caseloads and workloads of staff closely and frequently and ensure appropriate support is provided. Supervision should also go beyond everyday procedural matters and help illuminate the difficult and sometimes confronting aspects of practice. Supervision can be a way of recognising and developing the personal and professional resources of the worker and celebrating the gains they make. The degree and timing of supervisory supports should also align with workers' level of experience, with employees who are new to the service provider initially receiving more frequent supervision.

Managers are not only supervisors—they also have an active part to play in building relationships with people with a mild intellectual disability and with their staff. The following example illustrates this point:

> Rita is the team leader in a program which supports people with a mild intellectual disability to come together and collectively advocate for change on the issues that matter for them. Rita regularly drops in on the group to make herself known and chat to group members. Michael, a man with a mild intellectual disability and autism has been having a difficult time with his employment service provider and is becoming increasingly frustrated. He acts aggressively with another group member. The group facilitator is able to call on Rita to talk to Michael separately. Rita is able to de-escalate Michael's behaviour and talk through with him what triggered his behaviour and what is acceptable within the group setting. While Michael is angry initially, Rita is a familiar face, and he therefore can accept her intervention and her authority.

Rita's approach here illustrates how team leaders can support both staff and people with a mild intellectual disability. Her active presence in the daily work of the programme was beneficial to the well-being of all in the group, but also provided assistance to the group facilitator by managing the critical incident and modelling effective practice. Rita's involvement prevented the risk of relationship rupture between Michael and the group facilitator and allowed Michael to continue to feel safe and supported within the group. Managers within a relationship-based model have a primary task "to promote the effectiveness of practitioners and ultimately enhance the well-being of service users" (Ruch, 2012, p. 1329).

Organisational practices such as those described above do not occur in a vacuum. Practitioners and service providers must collaborate with outside service systems, and energy must be given to optimise these relationships and coordinate the supports for people with a mild intellectual disability. In addition, service models which include key worker roles and a team commitment to each service user can be particularly challenging within the current funding parameters of the NDIS. This may involve cross-subsidising the key worker model from other related programmes and identifying alternative sources of funds that can be used (such as project-based funding). The need to be creative, to forge helpful partnerships with other stakeholders, and to advocate for systemic change are all vital ingredients to ensure the survival of relationship-based practice. These issues are discussed in the next section on related service systems.

Relationship-Based Practice at the Service Systems Level

People with a mild intellectual disability are often high-frequency users of a diverse range of welfare services (Dowse et al., 2016). This multi-agency involvement in a person's life can create many challenges, especially when each service system responds to concerns in different ways and there is a lack of communication between service providers. Sarah's experience illustrates this:

> Sarah grew up in a chaotic family environment and from 11 years was engaged in high risk and illegal behaviour. As she grew older, she constantly sought out relationships with older men but these men sexually exploited her. More recently, she became involved with two men in their 30 s and 40 s who coerced her into sex work. They supplied her with methamphetamine, and she was trapped in a cycle of debt to these men. She also presented to hospital with drug-induced psychosis. The health system regards the issue as a mental health concern. The police see the issue as a criminal matter resulting from Sarah's own choices. The NDIS is focused on Sarah's intellectual disability. These systems can operate in silos and only address one aspect of Sarah's life. The key worker involved in supporting Sarah needs to understand what is happening to Sarah from a holistic lens. By building an effective and supportive relationship with Sarah, the key worker can be the communicative bridge between different service systems and can assist Sarah to navigate these supports in her life.

As indicated by Sarah's story above, each professional may have only a partial understanding of the person's needs, undermining a core human need of the person with an intellectual disability to be known and understood. Without overarching coordination of supports, a person with a mild intellectual disability may frequently move from one service to another, important information can be lost, and the frequent interaction with different professionals can become destabilising (Ellem et al., 2020).

The relationship-based practitioner fulfils a crucial role in helping the person with a mild intellectual disability to access supports from other service providers by maintaining a holistic perspective on the person's life, brokering information to these other supports, and mediating when conflicts may arise. The worker can provide important background knowledge about a person's life, their communicative processes, and behavioural presentation. They can also challenge any false assumptions regarding mild intellectual disability held by other professionals who may have little experience in the disability sector. A practitioner therefore needs to not only build a supportive relationship with the person with a mild intellectual disability but also create connections with stakeholders in other service systems, developing multi- and cross-system expertise (Dowse et al., 2016).

Cross-agency work can be fraught with complexity. To act with fidelity to the service user with a mild intellectual disability, a worker may need to educate and sometimes challenge other services which place too many preconditions on supporting the person (Ellem et al., 2019). In such conflicts, the worker must tread carefully, particularly if the other service is the only one of its kind available in the area. The cost to the individual person with an intellectual disability, to other service users who may want to access the service, and to the ongoing organisational relationship with the said service must all be considered. Workers must therefore be skilled not only in relationship-building but in respectful negotiation, conflict resolution, and advocacy. This reiterates the importance of organisations prioritising the appointment of qualified key workers to engage in this work, who have tertiary training in social work, psychology, or other helping professions. Unfortunately, such standards for worker qualifications are not mandatory or even encouraged within the current NDIS funding system.

Another tension is the competition between services for scarce funding resources. Many service providers are required to compete for the same pool of government funding, and this in turn can lead to the withholding of information and lack of collaboration (Haight et al., 2014). Systemic change, such as memorandums of understanding between systems, policy alignment between Government Departments on issues of concern, and creative ways of collaborating such as sharing resources, programmes, or interventions across service providers are all needed to provide the appropriate environment for relationship-based work. Collaboration can include joint applications for funding via consortium models to leverage the knowledge and skills of multiple service providers to meet the needs of this cohort. Without these overarching mechanisms, individual practitioners may expend unnecessary energy in negotiating supports for people with a mild intellectual disability with other sectors (Ellem et al., 2019).

Many of the elements of practice discussed in this chapter are predicated on investments by governments to consider the well-being of people with a mild intellectual disability, to draw on knowledge about evidence-informed practice, and to commit to addressing people's needs at a pace that suits each individual person. The NDIS is one such attempt to offer people with disability, their families, and carers greater choice and control over their lives. Its introduction across Australia has shifted the delivery of disability supports to individualised funding for each person with a disability admitted to the scheme. Unfortunately, the transition to self-direction has not occurred with concomitant attention to disability workforce training, skills, and remuneration, which is conducive to relationship-based practice (Cortis et al., 2017). Pricing arrangements for disability support work do not adequately recognise the need for supervision, development, and coordination activities for staff. In addition, there is significant unfunded work that disability workers do to assist people with a mild intellectual disability to access the NDIS and to understand and utilise their NDIS plans, as well as an increase in administrative demands for service providers to ensure quality and safety assurance (Carey & Malbon, 2021).

Many of the challenges associated with the NDIS model are beyond the capacity of individual service providers to address and require systemic advocacy over a concerted period. To support relationship-based practice, service providers need to build allies with other organisations to form a collective voice about issues that matter. Consideration of alternative sources of funding may also supplement relationship-based work, such as applying for grants for project-based work (such as group programmes) and applying to community-based and philanthropic funding schemes.

Conclusion

This chapter has focused on the positive impact that relationship-based practice can make in the lives of people with a mild intellectual disability, a group who are often poorly serviced by both mainstream and disability services. Relationship-based practice is based on reciprocity and prioritises the development of authentic, trusting, and supportive relationships. Such relationships provide the person with a mild intellectual disability a platform from which they can access support and build connections and confidence in order to take control of their own life decisions. To facilitate such outcomes, relationship work must extend beyond the person with an intellectual disability, to also include their personal networks, and the services and systems which the person encounters. Importantly, relationship-based practice is not about prescriptive interventions or 'techniques', but rather the quality of the relationship that is developed. To do this work, practitioners require a diverse skill set that spans micro, meso (middle), and macro practice. As showcased in the case studies embedded in this chapter, this may include, but is not limited to, skills in interpersonal communication, groupwork, negotiation, community education, and advocacy. Relationship-based practice of this nature requires significant commitment, creativity, and resourcing by both individual workers and their employing organisations. However, the dominance of individualised and market-driven funding models can constrain the ability of organisations to embed comprehensive relationship-based approaches into service delivery models. Thus, it is imperative that organisations actively seek to resist casualisation and de-skilling of the disability workforce in order to establish practice cultures that privilege relational practices and ongoing training and professional development.

Take-Home Messages

- Many people with a mild intellectual disability do not fit the box for mainstream and disability services and systems.
- Building authentic, supportive, and trusting relationships with this diverse group of people is paramount to bring about positive change.
- This relationship work extends beyond the person to their personal and formal networks, to the culture of an organisation, and to the services and systems with which the person comes into contact.

References

Anderson, S., & Bigby, C. (2017). Self-advocacy as a means to positive identities for people with intellectual disability: 'We just help them, be them really'. *Journal of Applied Research in Intellectual Disabilities, 30*(1), 109–120. https://doi.org/10.1111/jar.12223

Caouette, M., Lachapelle, Y., Moreau, J., & Lussier-Desrochers, D. (2018). Descriptive study of caseworkers' practices to support the development of self-determination of adults with intellectual disabilities. *Journal of Policy and Practice in Intellectual Disabilities, 15*(1), 4–11. https://doi.org/10.1111/jppi.12217

Carey, G., & Malbon, E. (2021). Implementation challenges in the NDIS. In M. Cowden & C. McCullagh (Eds.), *National Disability Insurance Scheme*. Springer.

Collings, S., Dew, A., & Dowse, L. (2015). *Being a planner with a person with disability and complex support needs: Planning resource kit.*

Cortis, N., Macdonald, F., Davidson, B., & Bentham, E. (2017). *Reasonable, necessary and valued: Pricing disability services for quality support and decent jobs.* Social Policy Research Centre, UNSW Sydney.

Dowse, L., Dew, A., Sewell, A., & CB/AH, S. N. F. (2019). Background paper for ASID position statement on intellectual disability and complex support needs. *Research and Practice in Intellectual and Developmental Disabilities, 6*(1), 5–13. https://doi.org/10.1080/23297018.2019.1594347

Dowse, L., Wiese, M., & Smith, L. (2016). Workforce issues in the Australian National Disability Insurance Scheme: Complex support needs ready? *Research and Practice in Intellectual and Developmental Disabilities, 3*(1), 54–64. https://doi.org/10.1080/23297018.2016.1161542

Ellem, K. (2019). Supporting people with cognitive disabilities in contact with the criminal justice system: The importance of relationship-based practice. *Research and Practice in Intellectual and Developmental Disabilities, 6*(2), 164–177. https://doi.org/10.1080/23297018.2019.1629332

Ellem, K., Baidawi, S., Dowse, L., & Smith, L. (2019). Services to young people with complex support needs in rural and regional Australia: Beyond a metro-centric response. *Children and Youth Services Review, 99*(Apr 2019), 97–106. https://doi.org/10.1016/j.childyouth.2019.01.033

Ellem, K., Harris, P., & Strnadová, I. (2022). Emerging from the shadows: Digital stories of self-advocates with intellectual disabilities. *Journal of Policy and Practice in Intellectual Disabilities, 19*(4), 360–369. https://doi.org/10.1111/jppi.12426

Ellem, K., O'Connor, M., Wilson, J., & Williams, S. (2013). Social work with marginalised people who have a mild or borderline intellectual disability: Practicing gentleness and encouraging Hope. *Australian Social Work, 66*(1), 56–71. https://doi.org/10.1080/0312407X.2012.710244

Ellem, K., Smith, L., Baidawi, S., McGhee, A., & Dowse, L. (2020). Transcending the professional–client divide: Supporting young people with complex support needs through transitions. *Child and Adolescent Social Work Journal, 37*(2), 109–122. https://doi.org/10.1007/s10560-020-00651-x

Grymonprez, H., Roose, R., & Roets, G. (2017). Outreach social work: From managing access to practices of accessibility. *European Journal of Social Work, 20*(4), 461–471. https://doi.org/10.1080/13691457.2016.1255589

Haight, W. L., Bidwell, L. N., Marshall, J. M., & Khatiwoda, P. (2014). Implementing the crossover youth practice model in diverse contexts: Child welfare and juvenile justice professionals' experiences of multisystem collaborations. *Children and Youth Services Review, 39*, 91–100. https://doi.org/10.1016/j.childyouth.2014.02.001

Healy, K. (2018). *The skilled communicator in social work: The art and science of communication in practice*. Palgrave.

McConnell, D., Feldman, M., Aunos, M., Pacheco, L., Savage, A., Hahn, L., Dube, C., Chenier, S., & Park, E. (2016). Ameliorating psychosocial risk among mothers with intellectual impairment. *Community Mental Health Journal, 52*(8), 944–953. https://doi.org/10.1007/s10597-015-9979-9

McManus, S., Ali, A., Bebbington, P., Brugha, T., Cooper, C., Rai, D., Saunders, C., Strydrom, A., & Hassiotis, A. (2018). *Inequalities in health and service use among people with borderline intellectual impairment*. NatCen.

McMaster, K. (2016). Social change through group work. In J. Maidment & R. Egan (Eds.), *Practice skills in social work and welfare : More than just common sense* (3rd ed., p. 261). Allen & Unwin.

Rasmussen, B., & Mishna, F. (2018). The process of facilitating case formulations in relational clinical supervision. *Clinical Social Work Journal, 46*(4), 281–288. https://doi.org/10.1007/s10615-018-0662-9

Renehan, E., Goeman, D., & Koch, S. (2017). Development of an optimised key worker framework for people with dementia, their family and caring unit living in the community. *BMC Health Services Research, 17*(1), 501–501. https://doi.org/10.1186/s12913-017-2448-0

Robinson, S., Fisher, K. R., Graham, A., Ikäheimo, H., Johnson, K., & Rozengarten, T. (2022). Recasting 'harm' in support: Misrecognition between people with intellectual disability and paid workers. *Disability and Society* (ahead-of-print), 1–22. https://doi.org/10.1080/09687599.2022.2029357.

Ruch, G. (2012). Where have all the feelings gone? Developing reflective and relationship-based Management in Child-Care Social Work. *The British Journal of Social Work, 42*(7), 1315–1332. https://doi.org/10.1093/bjsw/bcr134

Wieland, J., & Zitman, F. G. (2016). It is time to bring borderline intellectual functioning back into the main fold of classification systems. *BJPsych Bull, 40*(4), 204–206. https://doi.org/10.1192/pb.bp.115.051490

Wilson, N. J., Jaques, H., Johnson, A., & Brotherton, M. L. (2017). From social exclusion to supported inclusion: Adults with intellectual disability discuss their lived experiences of a structured social group. *Journal of Applied Research in Intellectual Disabilities, 30*(5), 847–858. https://doi.org/10.1111/jar.12275

CHAPTER 7

Supporting Engagement in Everyday Life at Home and in the Community: Active Support

Christine Bigby

Individualised funding is a primary mechanism for ensuring people with disabilities can access the individual support they need to have a good quality of life. Schemes such as the Australian National Disability Insurance Scheme (NDIS) enable eligible people to purchase support from the providers they choose. Such schemes have been most successful for people with resourceful social networks, who are able to advocate for themselves and direct their own support (Mavromaras et al., 2018). They have been less beneficial for people with intellectual disabilities, many of whom do not have strong informal networks and rely on others to assist in exercising choice and directing their support. For this group the quality of paid support is critical to their engagement in everyday life and their physical, social, emotional, and intellectual development.

Ten years of individualised funding in Australia has changed little for some of the estimated 25,000 adults with intellectual disabilities who live

C. Bigby (✉)
Living with Disability Research Centre, La Trobe University, Melbourne, VIC, Australia
e-mail: C.Bigby@latrobe.edu.au

C. Bigby, A. Hough (eds.), *Disability Practice*,
https://doi.org/10.1007/978-981-99-6143-6_7

in shared supported accommodation services (group homes) with four or five other people. Most are unlikely to have chosen their accommodation, the people they share their home with, their service provider or support workers. Many experience a poor quality of life without the skilled support they need to be engaged in everyday activities at home or in the community. Their lack of engagement means they have minimal opportunities for individual development or exercising control.

Despite the 24-hour presence of staff, some people living in group homes spend most of their waking hours disengaged—doing nothing. For example, an Australian study found that people with severe intellectual disabilities were engaged for between 0% and 57% of their time and those with milder intellectual disabilities for between 3% and 95% (Bigby et al., 2019). Indeed 52% of the sample received no assistance to be engaged, and only 9% received assistance for 14% or more of the time—the benchmark for good support (Mansell & Beadle-Brown, 2012).

Consistently it is people with more severe and profound intellectual disabilities—those who need more support to be engaged—who spend longer periods disengaged and who are less well supported. Below are snapshots from observations in group homes of people with severe or profound intellectual disabilities and their support workers. These and the other examples in this chapter are from unpublished data collected as part of an ongoing longitudinal study of the quality of support in group homes (Bigby et al., 2020b). All the names are pseudonyms.

> The support worker and the gardener provided some hand-over-hand support for Chris to hold the leaf blower and rev the motor and gave him some positive reinforcement such as "oooh, can you feel that?". Chris appeared overwhelmed with joy at being able to do it. This lasted a brief moment. Chris spent the next 10 minutes just watching the gardener from a distance, before he left the property. The support worker went inside and Chris was left alone in the backyard for another fifteen minutes before being asked if she wanted to watch television. She said "yes – cricket". There wasn't any being telecast that day, so the support worker suggested Chris come and assist with dinner. Chris was wheeled to the kitchen. For a few brief moments Chris was supported with hand-over-hand assistance to engage in the meal preparation. She was supported to place things in a bowl and hand items to staff. But there were many missed opportunities to engage Chris. For example, when the support worker was chopping up chicken Chris reached out towards him and was keen to be involved. She was told "no, you can't use the sharp knife I'm afraid". She spent a lot of time just watching.

> The two support workers on shift spent an hour doing paperwork at the dining table, answering emails, counting money and checking their phones. While this was happening, Scott, Joe, and Roger sat in the lounge nearby; they paid attention to the TV intermittently but spent most of the time just sitting and looking around the room. A fourth person, Josh, sat at the dining table, repetitively playing with his fingers. When the workers finished the paperwork they prepared dinner. While they were doing this Josh continued to sit at the table tapping his fingers or looking around the room. When the dinner was ready, the workers plated it up and brought the bowls to the table. One support worker sat next to Roger and fed him dinner while the second one sat next to Joe and fed him. Scott and Josh independently ate their food. The staff chatted to each other about their co-workers and other aspects of their job, such as their leave entitlements, while they were feeding Joe and Roger. After dinner, the workers cleared the table. One support worker washed the dishes while chatting to the other. Roger stood next to him and watched while he washed the dishes.

In contrast, some people living in group homes are engaged for significant periods of time and well supported to participate in activities and social interactions that are meaningful to them.

> The support worker sat on the floor next to Katie and read out loud the directions on the muffin mix box. The support worker asked, "Do you want to come and help me make these? This is what we are going to make" showing her the picture on the front of box. Katie showed no interest, so the support worker said, "I'll put all the ingredients in the bowl and you can help me stir, do you want to do that?" Katie's expression indicated she was interested but she pulled back when the worker started to help her get up to go to the kitchen. The support worker took the bowl to Katie and sat with her on the floor. She placed Katie's hand on the spoon, put her own hand on top and encouraged Katie to stir. The support worker said to Katie, "It's still a bit lumpy, what do you reckon?" and continued stirring. She asked Katie if she wanted to taste the mixture, and put some on the spoon and put it to her mouth. Katie initially pulled away, but when asked again she brought her mouth to the spoon and tasted the mixture. When the support worker said, "Do you want to taste some more?" and again placed the spoon near her mouth. Katie smiled and had another taste.

> The support worker was sitting at the table in between John and Janet, and assisting Janet to eat her breakfast. The worker noticed that John was disengaged and said to Janet "shall we put some music on for John". Janet

> smiled, and the worker said, "Yeah, good idea, eh". The worker turned on some rock and roll and said to John "There we go, mate, your favourite". John started to appear a lot more alert and gave a small smile. His physical appearance was changed for the next 15 minutes. At one point John started making a clicking noise, to which the support worker said "Are you singing?" He then clicked louder and began to make snorting noises too. All the while, grinning ever so slightly and rocking his head.

These stark differences in the engagement of people living in group homes are not due to the number of staff available but to the quality of staff support and their use of the evidence-informed practice of Active Support. Sometimes, known as Person Centred Active Support, drawing attention to individual tailoring and responsiveness of support, Active Support is an enabling relationship between staff and the people they support whereby staff provide.

> enough help to enable people with intellectual disabilities to participate successfully in meaningful activities and relationships, so that people gain more control over their lives, gain more independence and become more included as valued members of their community irrespective of the degree of intellectual disability or presence of extra support needs. (Mansell & Beadle-Brown, 2012, p. 14)

This chapter describes the rationale for the practice of Active Support, presents evidence about its impact on the quality of life of people with intellectual disabilities, and lays out its essential elements. The chapter reviews evidence about the frontline managerial practices and organisational features necessary to embed Active Support in services. Finally, it considers relationships between Active Support and other forms of more specialist support.

Why Engagement Is Important

Group homes developed in the 1970s to replace large institutions that congregated people with intellectual disabilities together away from communities. Until that time institutions had been the only alternative for people with intellectual disabilities who could not live with their families (Monk et al., 2023). Much has been written about the dehumanising conditions and culture of institutions that were characterised by rigid routines, block treatment, depersonalisation, and social distance between staff and people with intellectual disabilities.

Even in poorer group homes the culture is more person centred and flexible than that found in institutions (Bigby et al., 2012). For example, rather than the shared dormitories of institutions, people in group homes generally have their own bedroom. Group homes offer opportunities to tackle inactivity or disengagement, features of institutional life that posed significant obstacles to personal development—if people are doing nothing, it is almost impossible for them to have any choice or control over their lives. Engagement, the opposite of inactivity, is a precursor to quality of life. For example, personal development is only possible if individuals participate in new experiences. Interpersonal relations and social inclusion depend on interacting with other people; physical health requires activity; self-determination relies on people having options from which to choose and choices being respected; and emotional well-being stems from participation and relationships (Mansell & Beadle-Brown, 2012, p. 39).

People with severe and profound intellectual disabilities need skilled support to be engaged. Without support they are likely to remain disengaged and passive, as they do not have the skills or motivation to generate their own engagement. People with less severe intellectual disabilities are more able to engage in activities by themselves but often need support to explore new experiences and expand their repertoire of activities, develop their skills, and participate in more complex or demanding tasks.

Engagement in meaningful activity leads directly to increased competence and independence of people with intellectual disabilities and indirectly to more respectful and positive attitudes from staff and others. Researchers in the early group homes demonstrated that when people moved from institutions they could be supported to be engaged for much longer periods of time if staff used the opportunities for engagement offered by the many household tasks that needed to be done in group homes—for example, cooking, shopping, laundry, cleaning, gardening. Their work suggested that staff in accommodation services should facilitate people's engagement in everyday activities and relationships and that.

> instead of doing all the housework as effectively as possible, and then attempting to occupy clients for long periods of each day with toys, staff could perhaps be organized to spend most of the day doing housework with clients, arranging each activity to maximize the opportunities for clients with different levels of activity to participate. (Mansell et al., 1982, p. 603)

The benefits of the time spent engaged in such tasks potentially outweigh the benefits from relatively short periods of leisure, community access, or therapy programmes delivered separately from group home support.

Significance and Essential Components of Active Support

UK researchers developed and refined Active Support as a practice for frontline workers to support engagement. Initially developed in the context of group homes, Active Support is also relevant for staff who support people to use public facilities, such as swimming pools or libraries or to participate in community groups, employment, or volunteering (see Chap. 4). A significant body of research shows the positive impact on people with intellectual disabilities when staff use Active Support. This includes:

- Increased engagement in meaningful activity and social interaction;
- Increased assistance from staff;
- Improved skills, personal development, or adaptive behaviour;
- Improved choice, self-determination, and autonomy;
- Reduced challenging behaviour; and
- Reduced mental health issues such as depression (see Mansell & Beadle-Brown, 2012 for summary).

Active Support is the only strongly evidence-informed practice for support workers. The benefits of its use are overwhelming. It should be the foundational skill set of all support workers who work with people with intellectual disabilities, as it is these staff who spend the most time with people and deliver the bulk of day-to-day support which influences people's levels of engagement. Active Support is the way support workers should work all the time: how they should provide support and how they should interact with the people they support. It is not something that is scheduled for particular times of the day or parts of their shift or only relevant to some of their tasks.

Active Support is underpinned by theory and empirical evidence. It brings together into one practice knowledge, values, and skills that are often taught separately. Rights-based values and knowledge about things such as task analysis, communication, behavioural reinforcement, and learning are translated into this specific person-centred practice that can be taught to support workers regardless of previous education and training. It is the responsibility of disability service providers who work with people with intellectual disabilities and their families or advocates to ensure Active Support is embedded in organisations as the foundation skill of all support workers and frontline managers (see Bigby & Humphreys, 2021, 2023).

Active Support has two components: the way workers provide support and the way they interact with the people they support. These are broken down further in Table 7.1.

These components are captured by the catchphrases of the four essential elements of Active Support taught in training (see Fig. 7.1). Each of the essentials are described below and illustrated by short videos in free online Active Support training resources (Bigby & Humphreys, 2023).

Every Moment Has Potential

There are opportunities for workers to support a person to be engaged in many tasks, activities, and social interactions that happen naturally during the day. Workers should be continuously alert to opportunities to support engagement. One way to do this is breaking down what might appear to be complex activities into parts and thinking about the various steps of the activity that a person might be involved in. A good motto for workers is never to do a task alone but rather think how they can support a person to participate. This might be anything from cooking dinner, going shopping, playing a game, to buying a ticket at the cinema, or ordering a meal. Creating opportunities for conversations or social interaction directly with the person or supporting their interactions with others such as family, coresidents, or neighbours is also part of using the potential of every moment.

Table 7.1 Components of active support

Ways support is provided	*Ways of interacting with the person*
• Offering real activities • Offering choice • Creating opportunities to be engaged • Giving the right type and amount of assistance • Ensuring the message is clear about what is being offered	• Noticing and responding to communication • Respecting the person in all interactions • Creating opportunities for friendly interactions

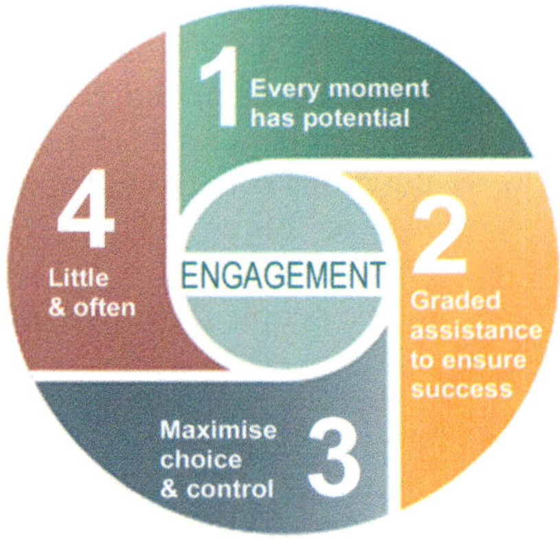
1
Every moment
has potential
2
Graded
assistance
to ensure
success
3
Maximise
choice
& control
4
Little
& often
ENGAGEMENT

Fig. 7.1 Four essentials of Active Support

> They unpacked Bridget's bag together. The support worker said, "you can pop these in the bin", pointing to the yoghurt containers and "I'll give this a bit of a wash", pointing to the dish. Bridget put some yoghurt containers into a bin while the support worker rinsed a dish in the sink. The support worker assisted Bridget to select items and pack her lunch for the next day, using verbal prompts for each step. "Do you need some fruit?" "Do you think that's enough?" "What type of yoghurt do you want?" When this task was finished the support worker chatted to Bridget about what she had done that day, and what was happening tomorrow. … A bit later the support worker prompted Bridget to find her bed linen that had been washed, asking her if she wanted to see if it was in the laundry. Bridget retrieved the washing from the laundry and began folding some towels and sheets in the lounge room. Bridget slowly folded the washing for about 40 minutes, while occasionally stopping to watch television or talk to the workers. While Bridget was folding, the worker began a conversation about Australian rules football. She stopped folding the washing for a while and together they looked at a printed calendar of AFL fixtures to figure out which games were coming up.

Graded Assistance to Ensure Success

There is no one way to provide support—rather support must be individualised, tailored to the person and the activity or social interaction. Workers must provide the right type of assistance for an individual to succeed. If they provide too little assistance or the wrong type the person may not succeed. If they provide too much assistance they take away opportunities for a person to participate or develop their skills. Ways of providing assistance include asking, instructing, prompting, gesturing, demonstrating, guiding hand-over-hand, or simply encouraging the person to participate and then standing back and giving them the opportunity to do it at their own pace.

> The support worker asked Kay if she wanted a hot drink or a cold drink, holding up the kettle and a glass as she did so. Kay indicated a cold drink by pointing to the glass. The support worker said, "okay, how about you get the milk out?" She prompted Kay by pointing to the fridge and saying "get the milk". Kay opened the fridge door and took the milk from the fridge door and put it on the bench. The support worker provided hand-over-hand assistance to Kay so she could pour the milk into the blender. There was a brief moment where a small amount of milk fell onto the floor, but this was met with good humour and reassurance from the support worker. Then the support worker held up two tins of flavouring and asked which one she would prefer, naming the two flavours as she showed her. After Kay had picked a flavour, the support worker pointed to the drawer and said "can you get out the spoon". Kay did so and then the support worker opened the lid of the tin with the spoon and supported Kay to scoop out some powder and put it in the blender. She gave Kay hand-over-hand assistance to push the button that started the blender.

Maximising Choice and Control

Workers must offer choices and respect preferences to increase a person's control over their life. Communication is important to offering choices and understanding preferences. Everyone has preferences but may express them differently, using words, actions, or facial expressions. For people to exercise choice, workers must offer more than one option. They might use words or gestures; show a person objects, pictures, or a video; or assist a person to have new experiences to expand their knowledge about what's available. Workers need to give the person time to communicate, check they have understood, and act on their expressed preferences.

> The support worker sat with Angela in the office and helped her plan a holiday. They sat near a computer and the worker talked to Angela about the various cities she could visit. Angela said she would like to go to Sydney. The

worker asked her when she wanted to go, saying "May, June, July, August". Angela replied, "August." The worker asked if Angela was sure she wanted August rather than May, June or July. Angela nodded. The worker asked Angela what she would like to do in Sydney, and Angela replied "go around Sydney." Realising that her open-ended question was too broad, the worker began to tell Angela about the different places she might visit, the Opera House, the ferry, the art gallery. She showed Angela a YouTube video of a Sydney ferry ride and they watched a video showing a range of Sydney landmarks. The supervisor then said the name of the landmarks they had seen, followed by "yes/no?" and Angela replied, indicating whether she wanted to visit that place. The support worker also used her knowledge that Angela liked to watch the TV show Sunrise and suggested that she might want to visit the studio in Sydney where it is filmed.

Little and Often

Some people can only sustain engagement for short periods, as they find it difficult to concentrate and need to take breaks. Workers should recognise this and support a person to dip in and out of activities as it suits them. They should ensure a person can return to an activity if they wish by avoiding packing up or finishing up an activity too soon.

Many people also need time to become familiar with a new activity before sustaining it for a longer period or deciding if they enjoy it. Workers need to offer new activities more than once to give people a chance to get used to them before making judgements about them.

The supporter worker was prompting Rod to use the tongs to turn over the sausages on the stove top. Rod enjoyed this activity for about 5 minutes and then put down the tongs and walked outside to the garden. A little while later the support worker carried the tongs out to Rod and said, "Dinner's starting to smell good. You want to come in and turn the sausages some more?" Rod did not reply and the worker said, "When you're ready. Come in when you're ready." After five minutes she went out again and asked if he wanted to come in and get gravy mix? You come in when you're ready." Rod came into the kitchen smiling. The worker commented on his smile and told him the gravy mix was in the pantry. He opened the pantry and when he seemed to struggle to find the gravy mix, she added, "Top shelf." He got the gravy mix from the pantry and the worker praised him, saying, "Good man."

Active Support is not only about providing support using the four essentials but also about the way workers interact with the people they support, showing respect and warmth and where appropriate using humour. Although not one of the four essentials, knowing a person well is important to the quality of Active Support workers provide. It is difficult to provide just the right amount of assistance unless you know a person's skills, or to offer and respect choices unless you know how a person communicates. Spending time with a person is the best way of getting to know them but may not always be possible. Workers can get to know about people quickly by talking to others who know them well; reading file notes, one-page profiles, communication dictionaries or watching quick video snapshots created through digital technologies.

Active Support is a staff practice, not a set of procedures to be learned or ticked off by workers. Good Active Support looks different for each person and each activity; sometimes a worker prompts a person to be engaged and stands back, and at other times the worker provides hand-over-hand assistance to complete a task. Working as part of a team providing support to a person helps to ensure support is consistent and information shared about their preferences. Imagine what it might be like to be supported to clean your teeth or make a cup of tea in a different way every day. The quality of support a person receives every day contributes to their quality of life: it cannot simply be put on hold because there is a new worker or managers have more pressing demands on their time.

Support workers can be trained in Active Support, but training alone is not sufficient; workers need to continue to develop their skills and work as part of a team in an environment where good Active Support practice is expected and valued. Creating such work environments is the responsibility of organisations that employ workers and deliver services to people with intellectual disabilities.

Embedding Active Support in Organisations

Australian research has identified the predictors of good Active Support practice, demonstrating the organisational features that need to be in place to embed it in an organisation. These are illustrated in Fig. 7.2.

Staff training in Active Support and their confidence in managers are important predictors of Active Support, together with the number and mix of people living together. Support workers can learn the basics of Active Support in a classroom or online training. They also need 'hands on

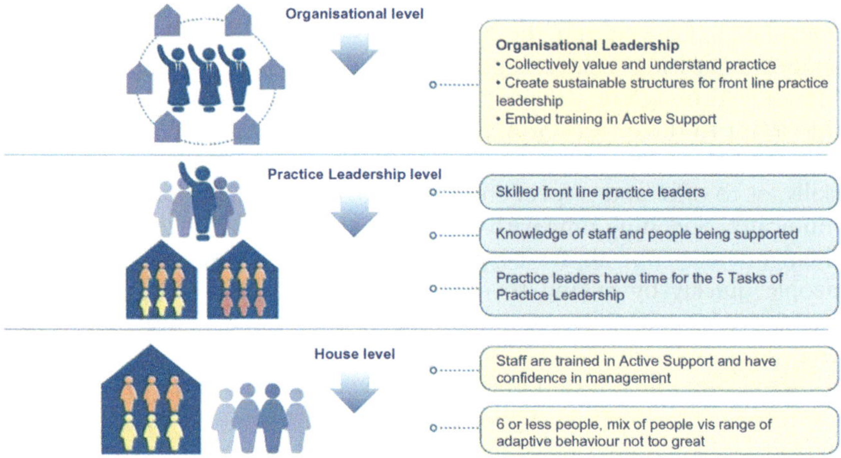
Organisational level
Organisational Leadership
• Collectively value and understand practice
• Create sustainable structures for front line practice leadership
• Embed training in Active Support
Practice Leadership level
Skilled front line practice leaders
Knowledge of staff and people being supported
Practice leaders have time for the 5 Tasks of Practice Leadership
House level
Staff are trained in Active Support and have confidence in management
6 or less people, mix of people vis range of adaptive behaviour not too great

Fig. 7.2 Organisational predictors of good active support

training' in their workplace with the people they regularly support, from an experienced trainer, to apply what they have learned to practise. Hands on training is important in assisting workers to tailor Active Support to the abilities and personalities of the people they support. Research shows people with higher support needs consistently get poorer Active Support. This suggests that support workers who work with this group find it difficult to apply Active Support and may need additional hands on training. There should be no more than six people living together in a house or one site, and they should have similar support needs. Other key predictors of good Active Support are strong Frontline Practice Leadership and senior organisational leaders who value practice.

Frontline Practice Leadership

Frontline Practice Leadership is a particular type of frontline management and is necessary to ensure good Active Support occurs all day every day (Bigby et al., 2020a). It is a set of five tasks incorporated into the role of front line managers. These are represented in Fig. 7.3 and described below. They are also illustrated by short videos in free Frontline Practice Leadership training resources (Bigby & Humphreys, 2021).

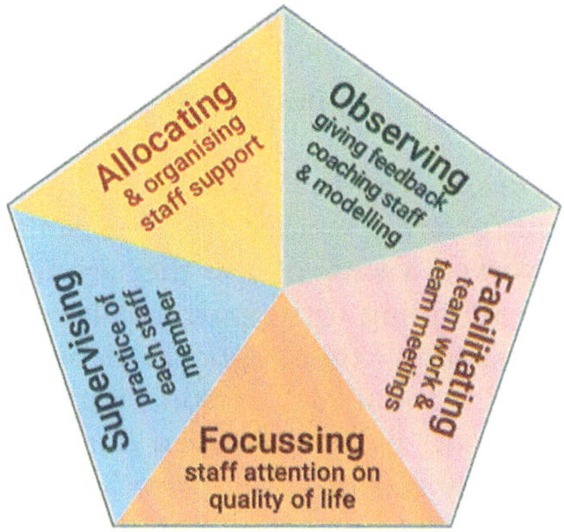

Fig. 7.3 The five tasks of Frontline Practice Leadership

Focussing Staff Attention on the Quality of Life of the People Supported
This task sets workers' expectations about their work, ensures they understand the concept of quality of life and see their role as supporting people to have a good quality of life (see Chap. 2, which explains the eight domains of quality of life). It can be challenging for workers to put aside their own preferences when they think about opportunities for activities or social interactions they create for people or the types of food, music, or décor they offer. Understanding the subjective nature of quality of life, that a good life looks different for each person, helps workers to focus on the individuality of each person they support. This keeps workers focussed on what is happening for the person and helps them remember that everyone no matter what their disability can have a good quality of life with the right support.

Supervising the Practice of Each Staff Member Individually
This task guides and develops workers' practice of Active Support. It is one of the most difficult and often avoided task for practice leaders, as it requires preparation, reflection, problem solving, and at times difficult conversations. It is more formal and lasts longer than the more frequent moments of 'observing staff, giving feedback, coaching staff and modelling good practice'. Practice leaders review workers' performance in supervision, giving them opportunities to reflect on their practice and discuss how it might be improved. Practice supervision draws on many generic

management skills—such as developing rapport, good communication, avoiding blame, and using open-ended questions—but is focussed on the quality of the worker's Active Support practice.

Allocating and Organising Staff to Provide Support

This task is not about rostering workers to be on shift. Rather, it is about shift plans that give workers a sense of how they are going to organise their time and whom they are going to support and how. Having a shift plan helps teamwork and maximises the support available to each person. Shift plans capture information about each person's regular pattern of activities and the sequence of events likely to happen during a day, such as what time each person normally gets up. They provide basic information about how each person needs to be supported with their regular activities, such as knowing that a person makes their breakfast but needs verbal prompts to do so. Shift plans can be written collaboratively, but practice leaders are responsible for keeping them up to date, ensuring they are used by workers to guide their use of time on shift and regarded as a flexible blueprint depending on preferences of each person being supported that day.

Observing Staff, Giving Feedback, Coaching Staff and Modelling Good Practice

This task is about continuously improving the quality of staff support. It gives workers opportunities to talk about their practice and get feedback about what is working well and not so well. This means that workers are not left alone to set their own standards for support. To do this task well, practice leaders need to be regularly present in services and spend time observing workers providing support. They should not rely on workers' own written or oral accounts of their practice, which are often inaccurate or lack detail. Regular presence in a service also gives practice leaders opportunities to actively demonstrate or model how to adapt the essentials of Active Support to the people a worker supports. Skilled practice leaders enable workers to discuss their own perceptions of their practice first and problem solve with them, thus also developing workers' own self-reflective skills.

Facilitating Teamwork and Team Meetings

This task is about sharing information and knowledge about the people supported to generate ideas for new activities or ways of providing support, sharing what works and helping to ensure consistent support from team members. Like supervision, effective team meetings need preparation and good communication. If run well, team meetings provide opportunities to review and discuss the quality of life of each person supported, share experiences and examples of good practice, establish consistency across staff practice by agreeing how support will be delivered, reinforce shared values among staff, clarify key expectations of workers, and shape team culture (see Chap. 13).

Senior Organisational Leadership That Values Practice

From research, we know that Active Support is predicted by the values of senior organisational leaders who set expectations about the importance of practice and create sustainable structures and processes for the tasks of Frontline Practice Leadership and staff trained in Active Support (Bigby et al., 2020b). While paperwork detailing organisational intentions are necessary, it has little impact on what staff actually do. Commitment to putting in place structures and processes for delivering Frontline Practice Leadership or organising training is more influential on practice than paperwork. Shared language and understanding of practice among senior leaders are important to embedding good Active Support. It leads to collective responsibility across senior executives, with each executive recognising the potential influence of their area of work on practice, from the management of finances and accounting to human resource functions.

Organisational structures should ensure that frontline managers have the time, authority and skills to create the conditions for teamwork and continuous practice improvement and to keep the focus of workers on the quality of life of the people being supported. Ways of structuring tasks of Frontline Practice Leadership differ between organisations influenced by the number of people supported in each service, the complexity of their support needs, the skills of direct support workers, and the overall management structure of the organisation. Job titles, span of control, and responsibility for other tasks may differ, but the pivotal issue in structuring Frontline Practice Leadership is ensuring those with responsibility for these tasks have time to do them well, spend time in services, and are close enough to the frontline to know the workers and the people they support. It is also important they have clear expectations about their role, and are supported and trained in Active Support and Frontline Practice Leadership.

While paperwork such as behaviour upport plans, medication records, or incidents reports are necessary, some paperwork more reliably serves its purpose than others. The volume of paperwork, both hard copy and digital, has increased exponentially since the first group homes were established. It is often seen by support workers and practice leaders as burdensome and detracting attention from practice (Quilliam et al., 2018). In designing internal quality systems and audit processes, senior leaders should heed the advice of researchers that observation is a more effective way of capturing and making judgements about the quality of practice than paperwork (see Chap. 14).

Dangers of Being Oversupported

As suggested earlier, skilled use of Active Support, particularly with people with mild intellectual disabilities, can mean support workers prompt a person to be engaged and then stand back, leaving them to start and complete an activity. If the right type and amount of assistance is not provided (i.e. graded assistance to ensure success), a person may get more support than they need, which takes away their independence. Being oversupported, like being undersupported, stifles personal, intellectual, and skill development. This is illustrated in the example below:

> Brian works full time in a logistics company. He is close to getting a karate black belt. When he arrived home, he told the worker he was not going to have the dinner with the other people in the house and would make something else for himself. After getting changed, he went into the kitchen and while the others were having dinner chatted to the support worker and scrolled through his mobile phone. He complained to the support worker about the processed meat in the meal she had cooked. The support worker, who had only met Brian once before said, that she could make him spaghetti carbonara. She made some pasta in a fry pan while Brain sat at the dining table, scrolling through his phone and chatting. When it was cooked, she brought it over to him. When he finished eating, he went into the kitchen, looking for the coffee. As he was spooning the coffee into the cup the support worker said, "No, that's too much…go and sit down, I'll do it for you". Brian went into the lounge and while he drank his coffee watched the news, commenting briefly to another support worker about one of the stories about the weather. Brian then went to the kitchen and loaded the dishwasher. He unwrapped a dishwashing tablet and placed it in the dishwasher. As he was heading to the bathroom to get his medication, the support

worker asked Brian to remind her at 8 o'clock that he needed to have his medication again. He told her that already had an alarm set in his phone.

Brian's situation exemplifies the way that well-intentioned but poorly skilled staff can obstruct a person with mild intellectual disability from being engaged in their own life. It also raises two further issues. First, the suitability of group home for a person like Brian who does not need that level of support. Evidence suggests that approximately 30% of people living in group homes have the same skills as people living more independently and do not need 24-hour support (Bigby et al., 2018). Second, whether Brian and others in similar situations are supported to consider alternatives to group homes. Individualised funding holds the potential for people to take their funding elsewhere and try other types of accommodation. Yet to make this a reality many people will need independent support to explore and make decisions about where they choose to live (see Chap. 11).

In Australia there are an increasing number of housing options, with differing levels of support available, where people can live alone or with one or two other people of their choice. These include, for example, single-person apartments scattered across one level in an apartment building which has 24-hour on-call support available shared amongst a number of people, drop-in-support for tenants in private rental or social housing, or separate single- or two-person units on the same site with support shared between units. Notably however, there is little research about alternative housing and support models, but it is clear that the quality of staff support and supervision (the use of Active Support and Frontline Practice Leadership) will remain a key factor whatever the model of housing.

Active Support and Other Person-Centred Practices

People with intellectual disabilities will spend more time engaged in meaningful activities and social interactions and have a better quality of life if support workers use Active Support as the foundation of their practice. Service delivery organisations are responsible for creating an environment where workers are expected to use Active Support, focus on quality of life, develop practice skills, and work as a team. Although use of Active Support is most common by staff in supported accommodation services, it can be applied to other contexts, such as support to people in their own homes, in employment, on representative bodies, or in community, self-advocacy, or peer support groups. Staff use of Active Support is also good for staff morale and thus potentially a bonus for organisations in terms of increased staff retention (Rhodes & Toogood, 2016).

There are strong synergies between Active Support, Support Planning (see Chap. 8), Supported Decision Making (see Chap. 11), and Positive Behaviour Support (see Chap. 9). For example, a goal may be a person is engaged in meaningful activities or social interaction for at least seventy percent of their time at home, a support worker's knowledge, gained from using Active Support, that a person enjoys cooking, might be information collected about the person as part of planning and contribute to discussion of a goal to develop cooking skills further. In turn, goals in support plans, such as moving to live alone, can help workers to think about the opportunities and experiences they offer to a person using Active Support on a daily basis (Mansell & Beadle-Brown, 2012).

There are strong connections between the strategies used in Active Support to maximise choice and control and strategies used in supported decision-making practice. These include, for example, attention to communication, listening and engaging, breaking things down, and creating opportunities to experience options and preferences (Douglas & Bigby, 2020).

Use of Active Support can reduce a person's challenging behaviour and their need for specialist behaviour support. As discussed in Chap. 9, the quality of services and use of evidence-informed practice, such as Active Support, form part of the system-wide and multi-component approach of Positive Behaviour Support. Indeed, some organisations represent Active Support as the base of a pyramid of interventions for people with challenging behaviour. Also, the findings from functional behavioural assessments conducted as part of Positive Behaviour Support can be valuable for support workers to increase the effectiveness of their Active Support by facilitating more targeted and precise support strategies (Ockenden et al., 2014).

More so than in the past, people with intellectual disabilities use multiple disability support providers. For example, a person living in a group home may get behavioural support services from an external practitioner, support for community access from another organisation, support coordination from yet another, and planning support from a Local Area Coordinator. Collaboration between professionals, workers, and organisations supporting a person is critical to optimising the overall contribution support makes to their quality of life. Good collaboration ensures that the knowledge built up in one organisation about a person is, with their permission, shared with others, and expectations about consistent support, use of Active Support, and teamwork by workers within one organisation are replicated by those in other organisations. Who leads or funds such collaboration is often unclear, but for those involved, understanding the synergies between Active Support, Positive Behaviour Support, Support Planning, and Supported Decision Making are useful starting points.

Finally, in the Australian context, from a regulatory perspective it is important that disability support organisations recognise that the essence of Active Support is included in practice standards. Demonstrating Active Support as the expected practice for delivering support across an organisation through internal audits or independent review will stand organisations in good stead for the formal audits required by the NDIS Quality and Safeguard Commission and give credibility to marketing claims of good practice.

It is not acceptable to argue that people living in group homes cannot have a good quality of life, that some people are too disabled to be engaged in their everyday lives, or that there is insufficient funding to deliver good Active Support. Rather it is the way staff resources are organised rather than their volume that makes the difference, and the evidence suggests it costs no more to provide good support than it does poor support (Beadle-Brown et al., 2021).

Take-Home Messages

- Engagement in meaningful activities and social interactions is necessary for people to have a good quality of life.
- Many people with more severe levels of intellectual disability need support to be engaged. For this group and those with less severe intellectual disabilities, good support can extend the range and complexity activities and develop their skills and interests.
- Active Support is an evidence-informed practice which can be used by staff as a way of supporting and interacting with people at home and in the community. Its use increases the engagement of people with intellectual disabilities, their choice and control, social inclusion, and overall quality of life.
- Active Support combines into one practice knowledge, values, and skills that are often taught separately, including rights-based values and knowledge about task analysis, communication, behavioural reinforcement, and learning. This specific person-centred practice

can be taught to support workers regardless of previous education and training.

- Active Support recognises there are opportunities for workers to support a person to be engaged in the many tasks, activities, and social interactions that happen naturally during the day; they must provide the right type and amount of assistance to each person for them to succeed, offer choices and respect preferences to increase a person's control over their life, and support a person to dip in and out of activities if they need to.
- To successfully embed Active Support in services, staff need to be trained both in the classroom and through hands-on coaching; they need ongoing Frontline Practice Leadership; and they need to be part of an organisation that values and uses a common language about practice and puts in place training and other management structures that reinforce good practice as a key part of its mission.

References

Beadle-Brown, J., Beecham, J., Leigh, J., Whelton, R., & Richardson, L. (2021). Outcomes and costs of skilled support for people with severe or profound intellectual disability and complex needs. *Journal of Applied Research in Intellectual Disabilities, 34*(1), 42–54. https://doi.org/10.1111/jar.12782

Bigby, C., Bould, E., & Beadle-Brown, J. (2018). Comparing costs and outcomes of supported living with group homes in Australia. *Journal of Intellectual and Developmental Disability, 43*(3), 295–307. https://doi.org/10.3109/13668250.2017.1299117

Bigby, C., Bould, E., & Beadle-Brown, J. (2019). Implementation of active support over time in Australia. *Journal of Intellectual and Developmental Disability, 44*(2), 161–173. https://doi.org/10.3109/13668250.2017.1353681

Bigby, C., Bould, E., Iacono, T., & Beadle-Brown, J. (2020a). Predicting good active support for people with intellectual disabilities in supported accommodation services: Key messages for providers, consumers and regulators. *Journal of Intellectual and Developmental Disability, 45*(3), 279–289. https://doi.org/10.3109/13668250.2019.1685479

Bigby, C., Bould, E., Iacono, T., & Beadle-Brown, J. (2020b). Quality of practice in supported accommodation services for people with intellectual disabilities: What matters at the organisational level. *Journal of Intellectual and Developmental Disability, 45*(3), 290–302. https://doi.org/10.3109/13668250.2019.1671965

Bigby, C., & Humphreys, L. (2021). *Frontline practice leadership*. Living with Disability Research Centre. https://www.practiceleadershipresource.com.au.

Bigby, C., & Humphreys, L. (2023). *Active support training resources*. Living with Disability Research Centre and Graystanes Disability Services. www.activesupportresource.net.au.

Bigby, C., Knox, M., Beadle-Brown, J., Clement, T., & Mansell, J. (2012). Uncovering dimensions of culture in underperforming group homes for people with severe intellectual disability. *Intellectual and Developmental Disabilities, 50*(6), 452–467. https://doi.org/10.1352/1934-9556-50.06.452

Douglas, J., & Bigby, C. (2020). Development of an evidence-based practice framework to guide decision making support for people with cognitive impairment due to acquired brain injury or intellectual disability. *Disability and Rehabilitation, 42*(3), 434–441. https://doi.org/10.1080/09638288.2018.1498546

Mansell, J., & Beadle-Brown, J. (2012). *Active support: Enabling and empowering people with intellectual disabilities*. Jessica Kingsley.

Mansell, J., Felce, D., De Kock, U., & Jenkins, J. (1982). Increasing purposeful activity of severely and profoundly mentally-handicapped adults. *Behaviour Research and Therapy, 20*(6), 593–604. https://doi.org/10.1016/0005-7967(82)90038-9Mavromaras, K., Moskos, M., Mahuteau, S., Isherwood, L., Goode, A., Walton, H., Smith, L., Wei, Z., & Flavel, J. (2018). *Evaluation of the NDIS*. Department of Social Services.

Monk, L., Henderson, D., Bigby, C., Broome, R., & Holmes, K. (2023). *Failed ambitions: Kew cottages and changing ideas of intellectual disability*. Monash University Publishing.

Ockenden, J., Ashman, B., & Beadle-Brown, J. (2014). Active support–fundamental to positive behaviour support. *Research and Practice in Intellectual and Developmental Disabilities, 1*(2), 98–107. https://doi.org/10.1080/23297018.2014.961528

Quilliam, C., Bigby, C., & Douglas, J. (2018). How frontline staff manage paperwork in group homes for people with intellectual disability: Implications for practice. *Journal of Applied Research in Intellectual Disabilities, 31*(5), 905–914. https://doi.org/10.1111/jar.12450

Rhodes, J. A., & Toogood, S. (2016). Can active support improve job satisfaction? *Tizard Learning Disability Review, 21*(2), 54–60. https://doi.org/10.1108/TLDR-07-2015-0028

CHAPTER 8

Healthy Lifestyles and Primary Healthcare

Jane Tracy and Teresa Iacono

Good health is important to everyone. Optimal health is central to being able to enjoy the best possible quality of life. No one can fully engage with, participate in, and contribute to their communities while in discomfort, pain, or distress in physical, oral, or mental health. For people with intellectual disabilities, however, sub-optimal health frequently occurs because of a combination of factors relating to their specific disabilities and external factors, such as where they live, who supports them, and challenges faced in accessing health systems.

This chapter provides an overview of the implications of poor health and why poor health is often experienced by people with intellectual disabilities. It then focuses on the role of disability support services and individual support staff in contributing to the optimal health of people with intellectual disabilities through the support provided to individuals and in

J. Tracy
Living with Disability Research Centre, La Trobe University,
Melbourne, VIC, Australia

T. Iacono (✉)
La Trobe Rural Health School, La Trobe University, Bendigio, VIC, Australia
e-mail: T.Iacono@latrobe.edu.au

C. Bigby, A. Hough (eds.), *Disability Practice*,
https://doi.org/10.1007/978-981-99-6143-6_8

interactions with the health systems. In this chapter, health is discussed in terms of physical, oral, and mental health as a whole because of the strong connections between them.

Implications of Poor Health

The implications of poor physical, oral, and mental health are far-reaching. Of greatest significance is reduced lifespan. People with intellectual disabilities in Australia die, on average, 27 years earlier than their peers in the general population and often from conditions that could be prevented if identified and treated early. They experience chronic ill-health resulting in pain, discomfort, reduced function, and hospitalisation and impaired quality of life at much higher rates than people without lifelong disability (Salomon & Trollor, 2019). People with intellectual disabilities also have high rates of dental or oral disease, causing pain and discomfort, difficulty chewing, bad breath, poor self-esteem, and chronic ill-health (Fisher, 2012). Similarly, rates of mental health problems in people with intellectual disabilities can far exceed those found in the general population (Whittle et al., 2019).

Distress arising from physical, oral, and/or mental ill-health is often made worse when the underlying cause or causes are missed. As an example, the onset or worsening of ***challenging behaviours*** (or ***behaviours of concern***) can be expressions of physical, oral, or mental pain or distress, but often is met with behavioural strategies or restrictive interventions, such as medications (Henderson et al., 2020). This response means that the underlying problem goes unrecognised and untreated, with the potential for it to worsen. Another possibility is that the wrong treatments are prescribed, which can create new challenges, such as dealing with the effects of multiple medications as new ones are prescribed to treat the side effects of each added medication (e.g. constipation).

Disadvantages Experienced by People with Intellectual Disabilities

There are multiple reasons for the poor health of people with intellectual disabilities, such that they experience health disadvantages in comparison with the general population. Contributors to poor health and health outcomes can be thought of in terms of risks associated with the person's disabilities (i.e. intrinsic to the individual) and those associated with factors outside the person (i.e. extrinsic to the individual). An example of intrinsic contributions to health outcomes are those related to specific syndromes and having a cognitive disability; examples of extrinsic factors include where people live and issues with health systems.

Intrinsic Contributors to Poor Health

Some health problems experienced by people with intellectual disabilities are related to their underlying disability, especially various syndromes. People with Down syndrome, for example, are more likely to be born with differences in heart and gastrointestinal system development (congenital abnormalities); the development and structure of the teeth, tongue, and oral cavity may lead to higher rates of oral disease; disorders of thyroid function may be present at birth or occur at any time throughout life, as can impairments of hearing and/or vision impairment. People with Down syndrome are at higher risk of gastrointestinal and respiratory disorders including gastro-oesophageal reflux disease, coeliac disease, and sleep apnoea. People with Down syndrome are also susceptible to the onset of Alzheimer's dementia at an earlier age than is typical in the general population (e.g. in their 50s rather than 70s); this onset can trigger disruptions to their lives and depression.

Because intellectual disability often occurs with other disabilities, such as cerebral palsy or autism, there may be multiple risk factors for poor health. For example, people who have cerebral palsy are susceptible to gastrointestinal disorders, particularly gastro-oesophageal reflux disease and constipation; dental and oral disease and orthodontic issues; musculoskeletal pain and fatigue; hearing and vision impairment; pressure injuries and skin breakdown; epilepsy; and anxiety and depression.

A person's intellectual impairment can also contribute to poor health through the impact on communication and ability to process new information, especially if it is outside their recent experiences or routines. People with intellectual disabilities vary in what they can understand and how they express pain or discomfort. Some rely on people who know them well to notice and report changes that can signal to a health professional possible physical, oral, or mental ill-health. Communication and related difficulties can increase the risks associated with some diagnostic and treatment procedures (e.g. having to undergo a general anaesthetic to allow routine dental procedures) and reduce understanding of reasons for specific treatments and willingness to follow treatment instructions. For example, someone with severe–profound intellectual disabilities may remove catheters during hospital stays or fail to remain immobile as required to allow wounds to heal.

Communication difficulties also impact health literacy, that is, the capacity to access, understand, consider, and use information of relevance to a person's health, such as public health messages in the media or following health advice by practitioners (Chinn, 2017). Health literacy provides the information needed to alert people to the need for preventative strategies, including seeking routine health screenings and making healthy choices each day. People with intellectual disabilities often do not have easy access to health promotion activities, including regular exercise or nutritional meal planning. They can miss out on health and cancer screening, healthy weight management, sexual health reviews, alcohol and other drug harm reduction discussions, and even vaccination programmes. Poor health literacy, therefore, contributes to poor health and, relatedly, poor quality of life.

Extrinsic Contributors to Poor Health

Where a person lives, who supports them, and the characteristics of health systems all contribute to a person's health, with problems in any of these areas leading to poorer healthcare in comparison to the general population.

People with intellectual disabilities often live in socio-economic circumstances that limit their choices and undermine their ability to access good healthcare, participate in disease prevention interventions, and make healthy lifestyle choices. Employment can improve these circumstances, and many people with intellectual disabilities can engage in paid work. Employment offers not only financial security but also access to social networks outside the home and a sense of belonging and contributing to community. Unfortunately, the rate of unemployment is high for people with disability, in general, and particularly so for those with intellectual disabilities (Dempsey & Ford, 2009).

Where a person lives also includes whether they live in supported accommodation, such as group homes, with family, or in their own homes. People who live in supported accommodation are dependent on disability accommodation service providers for day-to-day decisions that impact their health and for access to healthcare services. Family involvement in these areas will vary between individuals and over time. For some people living in group homes, responsibility for health, including access to healthcare services, can be shared across available family members and disability support workers. However, people with intellectual disabilities often outlive their parents and, as parents age, parents may have their own health concerns and as they move towards the end of their own lives, their ability to support and advocate for their adult children declines. In these situations, the person with intellectual disability will rely increasingly on paid workers in all aspects of their lives, including health.

Disability support worker training does not focus on this role of building and maintaining optimal physical and mental health, nor does it provide information about how to navigate health systems and work with health professionals on behalf of people they support. Training during induction and later when on the job may include only basic aspects of healthcare, such as administering first aid and medication. In addition, service users may have one or multitudes of healthcare plans, such as those for managing epilepsy, asthma, or eating and swallowing problems. The development, oversight, and monitoring may be by various health or allied health providers, with varying support to direct support workers. As a result, disability support workers are often poorly prepared or supported to care for people with complex health problems or those who are at increased risk of ill-health (Iacono, 2010). This leaves many support workers feeling unclear about their role and how to best support good health and access appropriate health professionals and healthcare, despite often being called upon to assume these responsibilities on behalf of service users in their care. In the following section, the specific roles of direct support service staff that align with their training and sector expectations of non-health-trained staff are described.

The Role of Disability Support Workers

Disability support services staff, in particular disability support workers, play a vital role in day-to-day decisions that impact a person's wellbeing. These include recognising and responding to possible signs of ill-health, accessing healthcare, and supporting the person during consultations. This role does not require disability support workers or their managers to have medical or health training or to be knowledgeable about a person's intrinsic risk factors (such as knowing that people with Down syndrome require regular thyroid checks). Rather, fulfilling this role requires disability support workers to draw on principles of person-centred care and advocacy and to have good health and mental health literacy as is expected in the broader scope of disability support. The discussion that follows focuses on the role of workers and providers supporting people in group homes, although some of the material also applies to people living independently who still need support with their health.

Support in Making Day-to-Day Decisions that Promote Health and Wellbeing

The extent to which disability support workers in group homes can help service users make good health decisions will depend on their own health literacy and understanding of how decisions made on a regular basis can profoundly impact health and, in turn, life expectancy. For instance, disability support workers may offer and provide foods considered to be treats or plan meals that may be enjoyed but have high caloric and limited nutritional value. Workers may lack an understanding of the importance of regular daily healthy lifestyle choices on physical and mental health. Unfortunately, poor health choices by disability support workers can influence those same choices by service users: for example, smoking while sitting in the backyard with a service user exposes them to the effect of passive smoking and provides a model a service user may want to follow. Disability support workers, with strong support from practice leaders and managers, require sufficient health literacy to support healthy choices and lifestyles that lead to (a) physical fitness and a healthy weight; (b) good hygiene, including oral and bowel health and menstrual management in women; (c) optimal independent mobility; (d) avoidance of smoking and substance abuse; and (e) bone and joint health.

Armed with this health literacy, disability support workers can help service users with intellectual disabilities to make good choices across the day that will minimise the risk of chronic conditions, such as high blood pressure and being overweight, which can, in turn, lead to cardiovascular disease, diabetes, osteoporosis, arthritis, muscle weakness, and low energy. Maintaining good physical health also supports mental health by increasing the person's ability and opportunity to engage in social activities, build and maintain social networks, and participate in and contribute to communities. People with intellectual disabilities require explanations, guidance, and opportunities to make healthy food choices, maintain a healthy weight, and engage in regular exercise to promote good cardio function and build strength. Evidence of the benefits of this support comes from a review of research by Heller et al. (2011). They found that supporting people with even severe intellectual disability to engage in community-based exercise programmes (such as fitness classes) and to make healthy food choices can improve their fitness and help them achieve a healthier weight. Psycho-social benefits were also found in this review to result from community-based exercise programmes, such as forming social connections and developing positive attitudes towards exercise. Important to achieving these benefits was help from disability support workers in accessing and engaging in these community programmes.

Responding to Possible Signs of Ill Health

Disability support workers have often supported individual service users over extended periods and know them well. This knowledge and seeing people in daily situations means that disability support workers are well placed to notice changes in a person that could signal health problems. Such changes can be seen in affect (being happy or sad), behaviours (becoming inactive or demonstrating challenging behaviours or behaviours of concern), or not wanting to engage with activities that would usually interest them or with people whose company they would typically seek out. These changes can indicate possible problems across physical, oral, or mental health. Direct support workers are not expected to know what the underlying problem is but rather to alert supervisors, managers, or family to the changes and to communicate them to healthcare providers.

Accessing Healthcare

People living in group homes are usually heavily reliant on their support staff to initiate, book, and support attendance at and follow up appointments with health professionals. The ability of disability support workers to advocate for and support access to healthcare will depend on their knowledge of the person's health needs, which is more likely if they have taken an interest in and supported them over a long period of time. Disability support workers with limited knowledge of the person's past and long-term social and medical history or who have worked with them for only a short period before being called upon to support their access to healthcare will need to collaborate with others. They will also need to have access to appropriate records, such as written observations made as part of health plans. Some general practitioners (GPs) will rely on structured strategies to ensure the person receives a comprehensive health check, such as through the use of the Comprehensive Health Assessment Program (CHAP), which has been rolled out across Australia (Lennox et al., 2013). The CHAP relies on collaboration between the person with intellectual disability, their GP, and direct support workers: structured observations of the service user and their medical history are recorded on a form by the direct support worker who shares it with the GP during a consultation. Responsibility for completing the support person's section of the CHAP can be shared with available family members, who often can provide detailed information about the person's medical history that may not be available to the disability support worker.

Disability support workers or managers must ensure that the person with disability sees appropriate health professionals for regular preventative care, such as physical and oral health checks, cardiovascular risk assessment, cancer screening, and vaccinations. Tools, such as the CHAP, which was designed to guide GPs through an annual health assessment, are particularly useful for those GPs who may be new to working with people with intellectual disabilities (van Dooren et al., 2016). Regular visits to healthcare practitioners can provide the care needed to achieve optimal outcomes for the person with disability while providing family and disability support workers with appropriate guidance to follow treatment recommendations at home.

Although disability staff or family may have responsibility for advocating for healthcare for a person with intellectual disability and supporting them to access it, adults with disability have the right to make decisions about their health and healthcare. Active involvement in decision-making will require assistance by family and/or disability support workers. This assistance may be in the form of providing and using educational material and communication systems or methods that reflect the person's preferences and abilities. Having opportunities to practise being active in discussions and decisions is essential to developing confidence and competence. Every opportunity to practise and experience the outcomes of those decisions, at first with small decisions and then building to more impactful decisions, should be supported and embraced. As with any new task, more coaching and guidance are required at first, with a focus on the short- and long-term implications of decisions.

Supporting Communication During Healthcare Consultations

Supporting access to healthcare includes supporting direct communication between a health practitioner and the person with disability which, in turn, assists them to be active in decisions about their health and lives. Healthcare practitioners demonstrating a commitment to communicating directly with the person shows respect for the person with disability as an individual and provides reassurance in situations that can be unfamiliar and even distressing. Disability support workers often experience healthcare practitioners bypassing the person with intellectual disability by directing questions and conversation to them. Their reasons for this practice can include the practitioners need to obtain information quickly and efficiently because of the time-limited nature of a typical consultation, being uncertain of the person's communication skills or unfamiliar with how they communicate, and general inexperience with people with communication differences. In these situations, an accompanying disability support worker can direct the practitioner's attention to the person to encourage the practitioner to do the same, model ways to engage and communicate with the person (e.g. through the use of signs, pictures, or simple but adult language) and to request permission from the person with disability to provide information on their behalf. For more guidance on this communication see Iacono and Johnson (2004) which provides strategies for GPs to better communicate with people with intellectual disabilities.

Healthcare Systems

Knowing about healthcare systems and strategies to work with them can empower disability support workers to advocate for and facilitate access to good quality care across physical, oral, and mental health for people with intellectual disabilities.

Designed as Mainstream Systems

People with intellectual disabilities access the same mainstream healthcare services as used by all other members of the community: this is true for physical, dental, oral, and mental health services. Although services are provided by professionals skilled in specific health areas, many will have had little training in delivering their services to people with intellectual disabilities. As a result, professionals, including GPs, dentists and oral health practitioners, and psychiatrists and psychologists, can overlook symptoms because they mistakenly attribute them to the person's disability or have difficulty adjusting to the person's communication needs.

Mainstream services, traditionally, have not been designed to accommodate the access needs of people with various disabilities, especially by applying universal design principles or knowing what and how to provide reasonable adjustments. Rather, the standard structures of the healthcare system, particularly in primary healthcare—GP consultations—often do not meet the needs of people with intellectual disabilities in terms of their cognitive and communication difficulties. Standard short consultations are usually insufficient to address communication barriers and to enable people to take an active role in the consultation. Enhanced or extended consultations can help address this problem, as can access to tools, such as the CHAP mentioned earlier, which is designed to assist healthcare providers conduct regular and comprehensive health checks (Lennox et al., 2013). Comprehensive annual health assessments and regular reviews are required to monitor and detect health conditions that are known to be associated with certain disabilities (those intrinsic to the person). Long waits to be seen by a health practitioner can cause distress. Noisy or cramped waiting rooms can also be problematic. For those who also have physical disabilities, lack of access to appropriate equipment such as chair scales, Hi Lo (adjustable) beds, and hoists can be further barriers. Discomfort, confusion, anxiety, or fear may be expressed through unusual behaviours which may further undermine the health consultation.

Working Across the Disability and Healthcare Systems

There is mounting evidence that physical, dental, and mental health services can meet the needs of people with intellectual disability when reasonable adjustments are made. Many health practitioners and health services, however, still lack an understanding of how to adjust to the needs of this group or are reluctant to modify standard practices. The principle of making reasonable adjustments is integral to person-centred care; indeed, it is a legal requirement in many instances. As the benefits and rights of patients to person-centred care are recognised, there is evidence from Australian research that healthcare providers are increasingly making reasonable adjustments for people with disability (Wilson et al., 2022). This greater willingness may be the result of changes in training, which, although not focused on disability, encourage healthcare practitioners to consider the needs of individual patients (Wilson et al., 2022).

Disability support workers, especially those working in group homes, and their practice leaders and managers can act as the link between disability and health services, enabling healthcare providers to make reasonable adjustments to ensure care and services for people with intellectual disabilities. They also play a critical role in bridging supports across families and healthcare providers, including GPs, allied health practitioners, dentists and oral health practitioners, and psychiatrists and other mental health providers.

Reasonable adjustments rely on knowing the individual with disability. This includes their personality, preferences, communication abilities and strategies, health-related activities, past healthcare experiences, and current and past health issues. Sharing this information with healthcare providers and ensuring the role and experience of family are considered can promote the collaborative process required for quality healthcare. The appropriateness and success of reasonable adjustments will vary between individuals and across situations. The following examples require collaboration across disability service providers and healthcare providers:

- Making appointments at times that suit the person (e.g. to avoid them missing out on favoured activities);
- Minimising waiting times by phoning ahead to coordinate arriving when the practitioner will be available;
- Requesting additional time (e.g. by booking an extended consultation) to enable optimal active participation of the person concerned and addressing all current health needs;
- Seeking and providing a low stimulus environment, including a quiet space with lowered lighting where the person can wait;
- Demonstrating how to adapt communication to the person's preferences and ability;
- Modelling plain language and visual aids for explanation and preparation;
- Advocating for time and support for familiarisation with and desensitisation to environments or procedures that may be frightening (such as vaccinations, blood tests, mammograms, or dental examinations);
- Requesting a plain language written summary of the outcomes of the consultation and any changes in management; and

- Arranging review appointments to check that interventions have resulted in the expected outcomes.

In addition to facilitating reasonable adjustments by healthcare providers, the following strategies are recommended for managers and practice leaders. They will assist disability support workers to fulfil their role in improving the health and access to healthcare for the people with intellectual disabilities they support:

- Require that, when possible, only disability support workers who know a person well accompany the service user to healthcare appointments;
- Set expectations that disability support workers support healthcare access, but do not attempt to direct it (e.g. by requesting specific medications from GPs or failing to comply with treatment regimens because the support worker does not agree with it);
- Require written records of changes noticed in individual service users, for sharing with healthcare providers (an example is the Depression Checklist, which is completed by support staff and given to the person's GP—see Centre for Developmental Disability Health, in references);
- Encourage disability support workers to demonstrate inclusive communication with an individual service user, which can incorporate non-speech modes of communication, for healthcare practitioners (see Iacono & Johnson, 2004); and
- Encourage a culture of advocacy, whereby direct support workers are encouraged to advocate for service users by (a) communicating concerns to supervisors and managers; (b) making appointments with healthcare providers; and (c) supporting the implementation of recommended treatments, including by communicating information about these to other disability support workers.

The example of Amelia below illustrates some of the practice-related issues identified in this chapter. It draws on authors' experiences as medical and allied health practitioners, as well as findings from their research. The example is de-identified and does not represent any one individual.

Forty-year-old Amelia lives in shared supported accommodation. She is usually active and socially engaged. She does not use speech but communicates enthusiastically using her body language, facial expressions, vocalisations, and photos on her iPad. Over the last few days, she has been unhappy and irritable and has been spending more time by herself in her room. Her support staff are concerned.

A member of staff took her to the GP, but her usual doctor (Dr G) was not available so she saw another doctor (Dr B) whom she had not met before. Dr B listened to the support staff express their concerns but did not engage directly with Amelia until he wanted to do an examination. He found Amelia had a slight fever, but as he approached to do a full physical examination, Amelia pushed him away. When Dr B tried again, Amelia got up and left the room. Dr B said he was unsure what was wrong, but prescribed antibiotics because of the fever and said to return if Amelia was not better in a week.

Amelia continued to deteriorate over the next few days. She stayed in her room and refused to eat and was reluctant to walk. The House Supervisor rang the GP surgery, explained the situation to the Practice Nurse, and asked for an appointment with Amelia's usual doctor. She saw Dr G two days later and was supported by a worker Amelia knew and trusted. Dr G spent a few minutes engaging with Amelia and looking at photos on her iPad. She said she was sorry Amelia wasn't feeling well and asked her if she had pain. Amelia's eyes filled with tears. Dr G asked if she would let her look at her tummy to try and work out what was wrong. Amelia's support worker and Dr G gently encouraged Amelia and supported her to get up on the examination couch. She was very tender in her abdomen and Dr G sent her for an ultrasound that showed gallstones. Amelia's favourite support worker went with her to the ultrasound investigation, and on the way home they stopped to get the photo frame Amelia wanted.

(*continued*)

(continued)

The lack of direct engagement and communication by Dr B led to a failure of accurate diagnosis and a distressing and potentially dangerous delay in treatment. The disability support worker and the doctor were not able to work together at the appointment to support Amelia get the healthcare she needed.

In contrast, in relation to the second appointment, the House Supervisor advocated for an appointment with Amelia's own doctor. Dr G engaged directly with Amelia, building rapport, trust, and confidence. Her disability support worker supported Amelia during the consultation to tolerate the examination. Dr G conducted a full examination, identified an issue of concern, and referred Amelia for an abdominal ultrasound. The Practice Nurse informed the disability support worker about what would happen at the ultrasound appointment, and they discussed how to best support Amelia through the process. A staff member that Amelia knew and trusted accompanied her to the procedure, and she was able to tolerate the procedure with the worker's support and encouragement. An accurate diagnosis was made which, in turn, enabled effective treatment to be provided.

Take Home Messages

- People with intellectual disabilities have the same bodies, the same health conditions, and the same right to good healthcare as all other members of the community.
- People with intellectual disabilities *rely on the same health, mental health, and oral healthcare services* used by everyone in the community, and these services are required to make reasonable adjustments to meet each person's individual needs.
- A proactive approach to healthcare is important when people are not able to clearly describe their symptoms. Anticipation of health conditions and the early detection of ill-health through the observations by disability support workers and family members is crucial for timely care.

- Direct support workers need to be observant of changes in the person with intellectual disability's behaviour, interests, or mood or physical appearance (such as a decrease or increase in weight or change in skin colour) and bring them to the attention of health professionals.
- Participation in health promotion activities nurtures healthy bodies and minds and builds and reinforces healthy lifestyles. Preventative health strategies include counselling in relation to the use of alcohol and other drugs and sexual health; managing cardiovascular risk factors; cancer screening; timely immunisation; annual physical, mental, and oral health assessment; and regular review.
- A collaborative partnership approach across family, friends, disability support workers, and health professionals, who each have a role in supporting people with intellectual disabilities, is essential to achieving and maintaining the optimal health, function and quality of life of people with intellectual disabilities. The common goal is to achieve and maintain optimal health and function and the best possible quality of life for the person.

References

Centre for Developmental Disability Health. (n.d.). Depression in adults with intellectual disability checklist. Monash Health. https://cddh.monashhealth.org/index.php/depression-in-adults-with-intellectual-disability-checklist/

Chinn, D. (2017). Review of interventions to enhance the health communication of people with intellectual disabilities: A communicative health literacy perspective. *Journal of Applied Research in Intellectual Disabilities, 30*(2), 345–359. https://doi.org/10.1111/jar.12246

Dempsey, I., & Ford, J. (2009). Employment for people with intellectual disability in Australia and the United Kingdom. *Journal of disability policy studies, 19*(4), 233–243. https://doi.org/10.1177/1044207308314946

Fisher, K. (2012). Is there anything to smile about? A review of Oral Care for Individuals with intellectual and developmental disabilities. *Nursing Research and Practice, 2012*, 860692–860696. https://doi.org/10.1155/2012/860692

Heller, T., McCubbin, J. A., Drum, C., & Peterson, J. (2011). Physical activity and nutrition health promotion interventions: What is working for people with intellectual disabilities? *Intellectual and Developmental Disabilities, 49*(1), 26–36. https://doi.org/10.1352/1934-9556-49.1.26

Henderson, A., McSkimming, P., Kinnear, D., McCowan, C., McIntosh, A., Allan, L., & Cooper, S.-A. (2020). Changes over a decade in psychotropic prescribing for people with intellectual disabilities: Prospective cohort study. *BMJ Open, 10*(9), e036862–e036862. https://doi.org/10.1136/bmjopen-2020-036862

Iacono, T. (2010). Addressing increasing demands on Australian disability support workers. *Journal of Intellectual and Developmental Disability, 35*(4), 290–295. https://doi.org/10.3109/13668250.2010.510795

Iacono, T., & Johnson, H. (2004). Patients with disabilities and complex communication needs: The GP consultation. *Australian Family Physician, 33*(8), 585–589.

Lennox, N. G., Brolan, C. E., Dean, J., Ware, R. S., Boyle, F. M., Taylor Gomez, M., van Dooren, K., & Bain, C. (2013). General practitioners' views on perceived and actual gains, benefits and barriers associated with the implementation of an Australian health assessment for people with intellectual disability. *Journal of Intellectual Disability Research, 57*(10), 913–922. https://doi.org/10.1111/j.1365-2788.2012.01586.x

Salomon, C., & Trollor, J. (2019). A scoping review of causes and contributors to deaths of people with disability in Australia findings. In: NDIS Quality and Safeguards Commission.

van Dooren, K., Dean, J., Boyle, F. M., Taylor-Gomez, M., & Lennox, N. G. (2016). Consider the support worker in the role of health assessments. *Journal of Applied Research in Intellectual Disabilities, 29*(6), 585–586. https://doi.org/10.1111/jar.12211

Whittle, E. L., Fisher, K. R., Reppermund, S., & Trollor, J. (2019). Access to mental health services: The experiences of people with intellectual disabilities. *Journal of Applied Research in Intellectual Disabilities, 32*(2), 368–379. https://doi.org/10.1111/jar.12533

Wilson, N. J., Pracilio, A., Kersten, M., Morphet, J., Buckely, T., Trollor, J. N., Griffin, K., Bryce, J., & Cashin, A. (2022). Registered nurses" awareness and implementation of reasonable adjustments for people with intellectual disability and/or autism. *Journal of Advanced Nursing, 78*(8), 2426–2435. https://doi.org/10.1111/jan.15171

CHAPTER 9

Supporting People with Complex and Challenging Behaviour

Laura Hogan and Christine Bigby

Different words have been used to describe the behaviour of people with disabilities that falls outside expected social norms and is harmful to themselves or others. These include behaviours of concern, behaviours of resistance, challenging behaviour, and abnormal behaviour. This chapter uses the term challenging behaviour, as it is most commonly found in the literature, while recognising that behaviours of concern is preferred in some Australian contexts.

Challenging behaviour is more common among people with intellectual disabilities than other groups of people with disability. As many as 18% of adults with intellectual disabilities display some form of challenging behaviour (Bowring et al., 2017). The extent of the challenging behaviour and the negative impact it has on quality of life highlight the

L. Hogan
Centre for Disability Studies, University of Sydney, Sydney, NSW, Australia
e-mail: Laura.hogan@sydney.edu.au

C. Bigby (✉)
Living with Disability Research Centre, La Trobe University, Melbourne, VIC, Australia
e-mail: C.Bigby@latrobe.edu.au

C. Bigby, A. Hough (eds.), *Disability Practice*,
https://doi.org/10.1007/978-981-99-6143-6_9

importance of designing services and developing practice skills to provide quality support to this group. This chapter defines and considers different types of challenging behaviour, the impact of the behaviour itself and how others respond to it, and its underlying causes. The chapter uses case examples to illustrate good practice. The examples are based on our practice experience and do not represent any one individual. The last part of the chapter reviews evidence-based strategies to support people with challenging behaviour to have a good quality of life.

The Impact of Challenging Behaviour on Quality of Life

Challenging behaviour is often seen as a person's way of communicating about their environment or situation. It may also be a symptom of an underlying health problem or genetic condition. Labelling behaviour as challenging can have lasting consequences for the way people are perceived by staff or services and should not be done lightly. Definitions of challenging behaviour convey a sense of its severity and seriousness:

> Culturally abnormal behaviour(s) of such an intensity, frequency or duration that the physical safety of the person or others is likely to be placed in serious jeopardy, or behaviour which is likely to seriously limit use of, or result in the person being denied access to, ordinary community facilities. (Emerson, 2001)

There are three categories of behaviour under this broad umbrella: stereotyped, aggressive destructive, and self-injurious.

- **Stereotypy behaviours** are the most common. These are repetitive movements or sounds, such as pacing, rocking, flicking, finger tapping, hand flapping, repetitive sounds or words, and walking in circles. While small amounts of each on its own might be harmless, when behaviours such as this reach high frequency and intensity they can severely impact a person's engagement in activities and relationships.
- **Aggressive destructive behaviours** are directed towards people or property. They include things like verbal abuse, physical violence, breaking or destroying furniture, bullying, screaming, sexually harmful behaviours, and faeces smearing.

- **Self-injurious behaviours** are intentional and often repetitive activities that cause injury or harm. They include self-biting, skin picking and scratching, consuming dangerous or non-food items, self-induced vomiting, or head-banging. This behaviour causes short-term pain and injury or permanent damage which can include physical disfigurement, vision impairment, or brain damage.

Challenging behaviour negatively impacts a person's quality of life, both as direct harm from the behaviour itself and indirectly through the response of service systems to the person and their behaviour. Harm resulting from the response of service systems means that much of the negative impact can be reduced by providing quality services and specialist interventions.

Denial of Human Rights

A frequent response by services to people with challenging behaviour is restraint or seclusion to restrict a person's autonomy or freedom of movement. Known in some service systems as restrictive practices, such actions may be sanctioned and regulated by bodies like the Australian NDIS Quality and Safeguards Commission. This Commission, for example, defines and regulates five types of restrictive practices. These are as follows: chemical restraint, mechanical restraint, physical restraint, environmental restraint, and seclusion (NDIS Quality and Safeguards Commission, 2020). The use of restrictive practices often compounds the negative impact of challenging behaviour and results in further psychological distress, loss of dignity, and autonomy and social inclusion. For example, chemical restraint that involves the use of medication usually prescribed for mental health conditions, to calm or sedate a person, can lead to psychological, neurological, or physical harm. However, it may also go unnoticed and unregulated, as this example illustrates:

> Jing finds noisy and unpredictable environments difficult. Every Sunday, the staff support the other people who live in her group home to host a dinner for their friends and family. Sometimes, the dinner overwhelms Jing and she calls people names, pushes them away, and slams doors as she goes to her room. Although Jing was not diagnosed with anxiety, when this behaviour started many years ago, her doctor prescribed anti-anxiety medication to be given to her by staff when the behaviour occurred.

Jing has recently had a new doctor who reviewed her medication. He is concerned that the anti-anxiety medication is causing a range of health concerns, including drowsiness and frequent upset stomachs. Jing has regularly missed work on Mondays due to being tired and unwell. Jing's staff were unaware of the side effects of the medication given to her most Sundays or that the practice was a chemical restraint.

Despite the regulation of restrictive practice, there is little data about its use. Dated figures from the UK suggest that up to 50% of people with intellectual disabilities in group homes are subjected to restraint or seclusion (Deveau & McGill, 2009). Longitudinal data from the Australian state of Victoria suggests that restrictive practices are often used long term and show that 74% of a sample of 1180 people with intellectual disabilities were subjected to restrictive practices for three or more years (Leif et al., 2023). Available national data about the number of times restrictive practices are used does not help to understand how many people are affected. Nevertheless, the figure of 688,163 incidents of unauthorised use of restrictive practices in the first six months of 2022 in Australia does indicate widespread use and raises questions about the effectiveness of the regulatory system (NDIS Quality and Safeguards Commission, 2022).

Regardless of compliance with regulations, using restrictive practices interferes with a person's human rights. Decisions about the use of such practices should reflect complex judgements that balance rights against each other, such as the right to freedom of movement against the right to be safe and free from harm (see Chap. 11).

Staff or service system responses to people with challenging behaviour, although not categorised as restrictive practices, may also limit a person's exercise of choice or restrict their social inclusion. In this example, people in Kenny's life made decisions that meant the loss of employment and relationships:

Kenny is a young man with intellectual disability as the result of the genetic condition, Fragile X Syndrome. He does not sleep well at night. When he is awake he repetitively bites the skin on his arms. This behaviour has happened for many years, and interventions have not been successful. Kenny has many scars on his arms which have started to limit how much he can bend and straighten his elbows. He used to work at a supermarket stocking the shelves. He enjoyed his job, was a well-liked member of the staff and lots of people used to pop by to say hi. Last year, Kenny's manager suggested he find a less physically demanding job. Kenny has not found another job and has lost contact with his previous colleagues.

Stereotyping

People labelled as having challenging behaviour are often stereotyped. This impacts their opportunities to participate in daily activities and in the way staff regard them. Staff may hear about a person's behaviour before their other characteristics, refer to a person as 'having behaviours' or temper tantrums, use labels such as 'grabber', or collectively refer to people as living in 'a challenging behaviour house'. Labels such as these stereotype the person as dangerous, frightening, childlike, or annoying and influence how support is provided. For example, if a staff member hears a person is violent with sharp objects, they might decide not to support them to cook, without being aware of strategies in place to support safe cooking experiences.

Disruption to Staff Relationships

The presence of challenging behaviour can disrupt the continuity of relationships between staff and the people they support. Supporting a person who frequently hurts themselves is emotionally distressing for staff. Staff who support people with aggressive behaviours may fear for their safety or experience physical harm. The emotional demands of working with people with challenging behaviours can lead to increased absences from work, lower job satisfaction, sudden resignations, and decreased quality of support. This example considers the situation of a female worker supporting adults with physically and verbally aggressive behaviour:

> Toni has worked at the same group home for several years. Two residents have regular episodes of aggressive challenging behaviour, involving throwing objects and standing over and yelling at staff. Toni has been hit by objects and bruised. All incidents are reported, and some emotional support is provided, but Toni feels that little is done to improve the situation. Toni is pregnant and is worried about her baby's well-being. She has taken a week off and is considering resigning from her role.

Reasons for Challenging Behaviour

Understanding the reasons behind a person's challenging behaviour helps select the best support strategies. The features associated with higher rates of challenging behaviour give some insights into potential causes. These include more severe levels of intellectual disability, specific genetic syndromes such as Fragile X, neurological diagnoses such as Autism or epilepsy, poor physical health, sensory impairments, boredom, and long periods of disengagement (Bowring et al., 2017). Challenging behaviour is unlikely to stem from a single factor but from an interplay of factors. Some of these are fixed and intrinsic to individuals (such as specific syndromes) while others are transient and associated with the quality of the support a person receives (such as the person's level of disengagement). This means some features can potentially be changed whilst others cannot (see, for example, Emerson, 2001) (Table 9.1).

Behavioural phenotypes are patterns of behaviour associated with other characteristics and specific genetic syndromes. For example, people with Fragile X syndrome are likely to have stereotypic and self-injurious behaviours (Langthorne & McGill, 2012), and people with Prader-Willi Syndrome to ask repetitive questions and have outbursts of temper (Oliver et al., 2009). The biological predisposition for such behaviours cannot be changed, but knowing if a person has a diagnosed syndrome is important for deciding which support strategies will likely be most effective in supporting a good quality of life.

Untreated physical and mental health conditions, which are common among people with intellectual disabilities due to difficulties of diagnosis or access to health care, may be the underlying cause of challenging behaviour. These may include pain, hormonal changes, reflux, medication side effects, constipation, sleep disturbances, dementia, or deterioration in hearing or eyesight. A sudden change in behaviour such as that described in this example indicates that the cause may be a health condition or pain:

> Daniel has a profound intellectual disability and is non-verbal. He started slapping his cheek after meals. This was new behaviour and staff thoroughly

Table 9.1 Intrinsic and extrinsic reasons for challenging behaviour

Intrinsic *Biological and psychological*	*Extrinsic* *Social and environmental*
• Behavioural phenotypes (see explanation below) • Physical or mental health conditions • Pain • Vision or hearing loss • Sleep patterns • Menstruation • Neurological conditions • Adverse life events and psychological trauma	• High sensory demands • Limited support for engagement • Inappropriate service design • Restricted rights • Lack of support for communication
Some can be changed	**Can be changed**

checked his mouth and gums during his oral health routine and did not notice any injuries. They booked a review with his dentist who found a piece of tooth missing from the back of Daniel's molars, exposing the nerve. Once the tooth was repaired, the behaviour ceased.

Environmental demands, such as high levels of noise or other forms of sensory stimulation, are difficult for some people to tolerate and can lead to learned stereotypic behaviours as a coping mechanism. An example of this is repeating the same sound over and over while walking through a shopping centre as a way of reducing the sensory overload of a busy and loud environment. Although this type of behaviour may not always be harmful, it may limit the activities a person can do or who they can be with.

Disengagement and boredom are also reasons for challenging behaviours. People with intellectual disabilities who live in supported accommodation with 24 hour staff support are at much higher risk of challenging behaviour as they may not get the type of staff support they need to be engaged in meaningful activities and social interactions. Services may not equip staff with the opportunities and support they need to learn the skills to create regular routines, communicate choices, offer opportunities, and provide the individualised support that some people require to be engaged. The absence of skilled support has a greater negative impact on people with more severe intellectual disabilities who find it hard to engage by themselves and whose communication difficulties make it difficult to seek out support in the way those with milder intellectual disabilities may. Indeed, in some instances, a person may learn challenging behaviour through the repeated and similar responses of others to their attempts to be engaged. For example:

Elly stopped attending her day program during the COVID-19 pandemic and has not returned due to staffing shortages. She is at home all day with limited planned activities and the staff are busy with administrative work and attending to house chores. They notice that Elly has started picking apart the lounge chair's stitching. When they see this happen, they sit with her, and talk about what is happening around the house. Over time, more and more furniture is damaged. The staff continue checking in with Elly, trying to distract her when they see her damaging the furniture.

In this example, staff reinforced Elly's behaviours by delivering positive outcomes in the form of social interaction.

Some causes of challenging behaviour are related to emotional or psychological development. People with intellectual disabilities are more likely to have experienced disrupted relationships with primary carers, maltreatment, or traumatic incidents in childhood than their non-disabled peers (Clegg & Lansdall-Welfare, 2022). If left unresolved such experiences may manifest in adulthood as challenging behaviours. For example, a person with unresolved emotional issues from childhood may become excessively attached to one staff member leading to aggressive behaviour when the staff member's attention must be shared with others or when they are leaving at the end of their shift.

Supporting People with Challenging Behaviour

For some people challenging behaviour is caused or exacerbated by the poor quality of services or other aspects of their environment. Ensuring receipt of good quality services and support is therefore a fundamental part of any intervention. This may be sufficient to reduce or prevent challenging behaviour.

Health-related causes can be minimised through timely attention to behaviour changes and preventative health care, such as annual health assessments and regular reviews by a person's general practitioner and other healthcare team members. Maintaining records of health assessments, recommendations, and follow-up are important points of reference to track changes that occur over time: for example, tracking menstrual cycles to determine the onset of menopause or regular cognitive screening as a person ages to identify slow decline that might indicate dementia.

Reasons for challenging behaviour related to sensory overload can be minimised by supporting choice about the types of places a person visits or the timing (going to shopping strips rather than large centres, or visiting early or late in the day when there may be less noise or people) or adjusting a person's home environment to suit their tolerance levels for noise or using equipment such as ear plugs or headphones to minimise the sensory load they experience.

Staff's use of Active Support as a way of working is one very clear strategy likely to diminish disengagement and learned behaviour such as Elly displayed. It is likely however that a combination of preventative actions by a person's everyday services and specialist intervention may be necessary to support a person with challenging behaviour to have a good quality of life.

Behavioural Strategies

Most specialist interventions for people with challenging behaviour are behavioural and apply principles from behavioural psychology. They use comprehensive functional assessment to understand the meaning of behaviour and develop multi-element support plans. Techniques such as Applied Behavioural Analysis (ABA) aim to understand and manipulate the antecedents of behaviour (what happened immediately before the behaviour), the behaviour itself, and the consequences of behaviour (what happened directly after).

Since the 1990s, the aims of interventions widened, to improving a person's quality of life rather than simply reducing challenging behaviour. This recognised that for some people the multiple or underlying genetic causes of people's challenging behaviour meant it was unlikely to reduce and that supporting social participation could not only improve quality of life but also reduce challenging behaviour (Bigby, 2012). Positive Behaviour Support (PBS) has become the dominant approach in both Australia and the UK. PBS is a whole of system, multi-component approach, that aims to understand the reasons for challenging behaviour and create change both at the individual level through expanding a person's repertoire of behaviour and in a person's social, environmental, or support system through redesign. PBS has twelve components which, as Table 9.2 shows, fall into three distinct types: rights and values, theory and evidence base, and process and strategy.

Creating a high-quality service environment, as well as individual assessment and support plans, is central to the processes and strategies of PBS. The next section turns to a consideration of assessment and support plans.

Assessing Behaviour and Developing a Behaviour Support Plan

Developing a behaviour support plan uses processes similar to those described in Chap. 10 for other types of plans. However, in this case the lead is taken by someone with expert knowledge about behaviour support. In some countries, this may be a person with recognised qualifications in behaviour support or a psychologist with specialist training. In Australia, the lead person is likely to be known as a behaviour support practitioner, who might have a professional background in psychology, allied health,

Table 9.2 Components of a PBS framework (Gore et al., 2022, p. 13)

Rights and Values: A focus on rights and good lives	1. Person-centred foundation 2. Constructional approaches and self-determination 3. Partnership working and support for key people 4. Elimination of aversive, restrictive, and abusive practices
Theory and Evidence Base: Ways to understand behaviour, needs, and experience	5. A biopsychosocial model of behaviours that challenge 6. Behavioural approaches to learning, experience, and interaction 7. Multi-profession and cross-discipline approaches
Process and Strategy: A systematic approach to high quality support	8. Evidence informed decisions 9. High quality care and support environments 10. Bespoke assessment 11. Multi-component, personalised support plans 12. Implementation, monitoring, and evaluation

education, or nursing or have no formal qualifications but is recognised as having relevant skills and experience.

The assessment and planning process should be collaborative, involving the person, their family or significant others, staff from their various service providers, and professionals involved in the person's life. A functional behaviour assessment is undertaken to understand the behaviour, its underlying cause, where it occurs, with whom, and what happens before (antecedents) and after it (consequences). This may draw on existing reports or new medical, dental, or allied health assessments to rule out medical or psychiatric causes for the behaviour. Background information about the person should be collected by reviewing reports and interviews with the person and key people in their life. It should include information about the person's strengths, support needs, their social relationships, and the services they access. Direct observation of the person's behaviour should also be conducted in the various settings where challenging behaviour occurs. Information is analysed to formulate a theory about the causes of behaviour, which then forms the basis for the development of strategies to prevent or reduce the behaviour.

During the assessment or intervention planning stage, reports may be sought from professionals with knowledge about specific types of intervention strategies. For example, speech pathologists can provide advice about effective and appropriate ways to improve communication, and occupational therapists can suggest how to adapt the physical or sensory environment or propose the use of adaptive equipment.

A behaviour support plan should include three types of strategies: preventative, proactive, and reactive.

- **Preventative** strategies aim to reduce or eliminate challenging behaviours. They include the types of actions discussed earlier: preventative health care, reduction of the sensory load of a person's environment, training and leadership for staff to implement Active Support to reduce disengagement and support participation in meaningful activities and social interactions, or specific psychological intervention techniques such as cognitive behaviour therapy.
- **Proactive** strategies are activated when a person becomes distressed, or something is happening, which could trigger behaviours. The aim is to intervene early to remove the trigger or provide the person with something they enjoy. Strategies may involve moving the person or others to another environment, calming, distracting, or re-directing the person. Remaining calm is essential to ensure the situation does not escalate.
- **Reactive** strategies are a last resort when other strategies fail to avoid challenging behaviours. They are used to gain control of the situation, cease the behaviour, and ensure the safety of all involved. Reactive strategies are often restrictive practices, such as physical or environmental restraints. They must be the least restrictive option available and used for the shortest time possible. Plans must also include strategies to fade out or reduce the use of restrictive practices.

Strategies must be practical and understandable to the staff responsible for implementing them, and plans must identify the people responsible for oversight and review. Where necessary plans must include details about the training and ongoing support available for staff implementing them and include ongoing data collection to inform a continuous cycle of review.

Psychodynamic Approaches

Some causes of challenging behaviour are related to separation or trauma in early childhood. If this is the case, alternatives to behavioural theories to inform specialist interventions are relevant. Psychodynamic interventions recognise the "untapped potential for development and growth in the emotional lives of people with intellectual disabilities that has the possibility to redress non-optimal life-histories and reduce distressed and distressing behaviour" (Clegg & Lansdall-Welfare, 2022, p. 6). These interventions aim to support staff connection with, and the co-regulation of, the emotional worlds of distressed people through careful "use of words, tone of voice, facial expressions, or body language that steadies the person who struggles to harness their chaotic emotions" (Clegg & Lansdall-Welfare, 2022, p. 6). For example, services in the Netherlands use a practice known as Triple C (Tournier et al., 2020). The Cs represent Client (the person with an intellectual disability), Coach (the support worker), and Competence (the activity which the client and coach perform together). This practice emphasises relationships, unconditional support to improve a person's attachments and relationships with support staff, to provide a secure base for joint activities. Several other practice tools to support practice-based or emotional co-regulation are described in detail by Clegg and Lansdall-Welfare (2022). There are, however, few professionals with this type of practice expertise in Australia with the consequence that behavioural interventions dominate practice.

Examples of Supporting People with Challenging Behaviour

The two examples below illustrate the service context and evidence-based practices, relationships, training, supervision, support, and teamwork, that may be involved in implementing a behaviour support plan and supporting a person with challenging behaviours to have a good life.

Joe

Joe is a young man with Prader-Willi Syndrome and moderate intellectual disability who lives in a group home with three other young men with intellectual disabilities. His housemates have similar support needs to Joe but none have challenging behaviour. Joe attends a community access programme. As part of his syndrome, Joe asks many repetitive questions and finds it difficult when things do not go how he would like. If the staff answer "no" to one of his questions, he argues with them. Occasionally, this escalates, and Joe slams doors and throws items within his reach. As part of his diagnosis of Prader-Willi syndrome, Joe has a range of health needs that require ongoing monitoring and review.

Services and Evidence-Based Practice

Joe uses accommodation and community access services and has a behaviour support practitioner. He also uses mainstream services, for example, a general practitioner and a dentist. For people like Joe living in supported accommodation it is not always clear who leads the coordination of their services and collaboration among staff. It may be a support coordinator or, in the case of Joe, the manager of his accommodation service.

The design of the group home reflects research that homes should be small with no more than six people and dispersed in the community (Bould et al., 2019). Attention has been given to knowledge about the compatibility of people living together, in that they should have similar support needs and people with challenging behaviour should not be grouped together. The organisations that manage Joe's group home and community access programme mandate Active Support (see Chap. 7) as the expected staff practice and it is embedded into organisational policies and procedures. Staff's use of Active Support to support Joe means he engages in meaningful activities and social interaction at home and in the community and exercises choice and control throughout the day. He is not disengaged for long periods and staff provide the right amount of the right type of assistance to enable him to successfully participate in household and leisure activities. Joe interacts with staff and people he encounters when he is out in the community (see Chap. 4). When people have choice and control over their lives and are engaged they are less likely to use challenging behaviours to express their needs (Ockenden et al., 2014). Knowing the person and understanding communication will ensure Joe's preferences are understood by staff and he understands the activities offered to him, which are important for good Active Support practice.

The organisation that manages Joe's group home keeps detailed records about his health needs, which are compiled into a one-page summary accessible to all staff. One staff member is his key worker: they are responsible for supporting him to attend medical appointments, interact with health professionals, understand their advice, share health information with other staff, and ensure all actions from appointments are followed up.

Relationships

As part of Active Support practices staff interact with Joe in a warm and friendly manner, treating him with respect and dignity. All the staff play an important role in his life, and he has a strong relationship with his key worker. These relationships, and the nomination of a key worker, accord with evidence that challenging behaviour is reduced when a central staff member is involved and there are positive interactions with all staff (Olivier-Pijpers et al., 2020).

It is not uncommon for people like Joe to develop close bonds with support workers. Aware that the turnover of staff can be distressing when staff leave, Joe's services aim to extend his social connections beyond staff. The community access programme he participates in supports him to attend several classes at a local recreation centre. One of the aims of the community access programme is that Joe will become known and recognised by other users of the centre and may begin to form friendships. Staff at the group home are aware of this strategy and support Joe to interact when he sees people from the centre in other contexts. Staff from his group home also support Joe once a week to use Zoom on his iPad to catch up with his brother who lives interstate.

Staff Training and Supervision

Joe's service providers are responsible for ensuring staff are competent and have the knowledge and skills to provide high-quality and consistent support to Joe. They have accessible and practical policies and procedures, an induction programme, training, clear reporting lines, supervision, and access to debriefing.

Reflecting evidence about effective Active Support training they ensure that staff have a practical hands-on component and theory components delivered in a classroom or online. As part of their induction all staff are given basic knowledge about Prader-Willi syndrome and taught about the procedures in place to support Joe to manage his insatiable appetite and constant need for food which are part of this syndrome.

Staff in the group home and community access programme are supervised by a Frontline Practice leader. Their role is to ensure staff remain focused on Joe's quality of life, get regular feedback on their practice and coaching to improve it. Frontline Practice leaders model good practice, support staff to work together as a team, and ensure they maximise their time on every shift to support Joe. This accords with evidence that strong Frontline Practice Leadership is associated with good Active Support and reduced challenging behaviours (Olivier-Pijpers et al., 2020).

The very specific strategies in the behaviour support plan developed with Joe and others will be shared with all the staff working with Joe. The behaviour support practitioner will take responsibility for briefing and training staff in its implementation.

Teamwork

Teamwork is critical to the quality of all Joe's support and successfully implementing the behaviour support plan. Joe is included in the team and staff work together with him collaboratively to ensure consistent support. Teamwork among staff in each service is facilitated by their Frontline Practice leaders, and a monthly meeting or conference call between leaders supports consistency and coordination of staff in the different services. This accords with evidence that challenging behaviour is reduced when there is cohesion between the staff team, collaborative input from specialists, such as allied health and medical professionals, supportive colleagues, and the space to make mistakes and learn from them (Olivier-Pijpers et al., 2020).

Sylvie

Sylvie is a young woman with mild intellectual disability, obsessive-compulsive disorder (OCD), epilepsy, and dental disease. She has moved to be closer to her sister and shares a unit with one other woman. She receives daily drop-in support to assist with cleaning, meal preparation, and to attend appointments. She has no regular activities but is interested in finding work with animals, making friends, spending time with her sister, and attending live music gigs.

Her OCD means she showers many times a day. In the past, this has meant she has missed appointments and scheduled activities. Excessive showering results in skin rashes and fungal infections. If staff intervene, she can be verbally and physically aggressive.

Service Delivery

Sylvie uses one service for drop-in support and support coordination. The support coordinator takes the lead and is negotiating a range of additional services, including a general practitioner with experience supporting adults with intellectual disabilities and mental health, a dentist, and a mental health professional to support her to manage the OCD and associated behaviours. Such services will be important to the success of her living situation as evidence shows that unmet medical and behaviour needs are common reasons that community living arrangements fail (Kim & Dymond, 2020). Accessing services to support Sylvie to find employment and social activities are equally important, as engagement will avoid boredom, help improve Sylvie's quality of life, and reduce her behaviours.

Relationships

The support coordinator aims to maintain Sylvie's relationship with her sister and include her as part of Sylvie's support team. Further the support coordinator will support Sylvie to find a service to provide opportunities for her to meet new people with similar interests to her own. The coordinator is also aware that Sylvie's relationship with her flatmate is very important. Advice from the mental health professional who will manage Sylvie's OCD about strategies for reducing excessive use of the shower will be important to avoid putting strain on this relationship.

Training and Supervision

The coordinator has ensured that the drop-in support service has trained staff about Sylvie's support needs and OCD. They have been trained in Active Support and take care not to over support Sylvie with household tasks that she can do alone with some prompting. She has also made the service aware that staff may need supervision and incident debriefing should Sylvie be verbally or physically aggressive. For staff working alone in this type of one-to-one situation, immediate incident debriefing is important to ensure accurate reporting, the well-being of all involved, and any immediate strategies to reduce the risk of another incident. Regular supervision allows staff who work with Sylvie to discuss support for her and opportunities for improvement.

Sylvie has a dated behaviour plan, written when she lived at home with her parents. Her mental health professional will update this plan and will also provide training for Sylvie's support team in implementing new or revised strategies.

Teamwork

As more services are established for Sylvie, training and sharing of information among new staff will become more important. New people will have to quickly get to know Sylvie and understand information about her support needs. The service coordinator will support the flow of information between these services which will help ensure that her team works collaboratively. Sylvie and her sister are critical members of this team, and an essential part of this teamwork is empowering Sylvie to be actively involved in decision-making.

Reflecting on the Use of Positive Behavioural Support

There are gaps in evidence about the effectiveness of PBS in the context of supported accommodation services (Gore et al., 2022). Some researchers suggest this is because what is regarded as best practice is seldom fully implemented in services. For example, one UK commentator suggested:

> It is relatively rare to find a service that has all of the recommended elements in place in the right amounts and combinations ....
>
> Most people with challenging behaviour still do not receive effective interventions even though adopting a positive behavioural support (PBS) model has been shown to provide them. Instead there continues to be an overreliance on inappropriate medication and restraint, the unethical use of control and punishment and exclusion of people from their own communities. (Jones, 2013, p. 5)

Data from the regulatory body in Australia points to the poor quality of behavioural support plans (NDIS Quality and Safeguards Commission, 2022) and research shows that plans are unlikely to be fully implemented (McGowan et al., 2017). Research also suggests that Australian policies misinterpret PBS as a set of strategies that narrowly concentrate on producing behaviour support plans and reduction of restrictive practices rather than a systematic approach to improving quality of life (Hayward et al., 2021).

A number of small studies do however suggest the effectiveness of PBS when external specialist behavioural services support accommodation staff teams (Lewis et al., 2021). Notably, in these studies, it is specialist teams that conduct assessments, develop individualised plans, and support accommodation staff with implementation. This suggests that specialist teams may be more effective than the arrangements in Australia where many such teams were disbanded as a result of individualised funding and replaced by sole behaviour support practitioners.

The largest and most rigorous study of PBS in supported accommodation took a 'setting wide' approach (McGill et al., 2018). Its principal aim was improving the quality of care and the support environment (see Table 9.2 Component 9) for people with challenging behaviours, while maintaining support from external behavioural specialists. Expected standards of support were defined, coaching was provided to service managers and staff to enhance their performance, and progress was regularly monitored. From this study, the concept of Capable Environments was developed (McGill et al., 2020). The study sets out the features that should be in place both in terms of the everyday support in a service and in the managing of the organisation to support a good quality of life for people with challenging behaviour. These are summarised in Table 9.3 alongside the evidence-informed practices discussed in this chapter.

This table may be a useful checklist for staff and organisations managing group home services or drop-in support for adults with intellectual disabilities and challenging behaviours.

The major challenge for organisations is to create and sustain the conditions necessary for supporting people with challenging behaviours set out in the Capable Environments framework. This will primarily be through the values of senior and mid-level managers, and organisational structures and processes they put in place. Culture is a key influencing factor on service quality and practice, and establishing a cohesive, respectful, enabling, and motivating organisational culture is a major task for leaders across an organisation. The nature and influence of culture has not been considered in this chapter as it is so significant that it warrants a dedicated chapter (see Chap. 13).

Table 9.3 Evidence-informed practice and services that deliver Capable Environments

Characteristics of Capable Environments (adapted from McGill et al., 2020)	*Evidence-informed practice or service delivery approach*
Everyday support	
• Support for participation in meaningful activity • Personalised routines • Support for communication • Support opportunities for choice • Positive social interactions • Support to establish and/or maintain relationships • Support for more independent functioning • Personal care and health support	• Active Support • Key workers • Shift plans (task of Frontline Practice Leadership) • Teamwork (task of Frontline Practice Leadership) • Staff focus on quality of life (task of Frontline Practice Leadership) • Preventative and attentive health care
Management and organisational context	
• Effective organisation context • Effective management support • Mindful skilled support workers • Provision of consistent and predictable environments • Provision of acceptable physical environment	• Frontline Practice Leadership • Supervision of staff (task of Frontline Practice Leadership) • Observation and feedback to staff (task of Frontline Practice Leadership) • Senior leadership values practice • Organisational structures for training and practice leadership • Small-size homes and not grouping people with challenging behaviours together • Environments reflect sensory preferences

Take Home Messages

- Challenging behaviours substantially reduce the quality of life for people with intellectual disabilities who display them.
- There are many reasons for challenging behaviours. However, some are easier to change than others.
- Challenging behaviours are more common for people with intellectual disabilities who receive accommodation-based support.
- Ensuring high-quality, individualised services and environments can reduce and prevent challenging behaviours.
- Specialist behavioural or psychodynamic interventions may be required for some people with intellectual disabilities and challenging behaviours. Implementing this requires significant collaboration between specialist practitioners and staff in services.

References

Bigby, C. (2012). Social inclusion and people with intellectual disability and challenging behaviour: A systematic review. *Journal of Intellectual and Developmental Disability, 37*(4), 360–374. https://doi.org/10.3109/13668250.2012.721878

Bould, E., Bigby, C., Iacono, T., & Beadle-Brown, J. (2019). Factors associated with increases over time in the quality of Active Support in supported accommodation services for people with intellectual disabilities: A multi-level model. *Research in Developmental Disabilities, 94*, 103477–103477. https://doi.org/10.1016/j.ridd.2019.103477

Bowring, D. L., Totsika, V., Hastings, R. P., Toogood, S., & Griffith, G. M. (2017). Challenging behaviours in adults with an intellectual disability: A total population study and exploration of risk indices. *British Journal of Clinical Psychology, 56*(1), 16–32. https://doi.org/10.1111/bjc.12118

Clegg, J. A., & Lansdall-Welfare, R. (2022). Helping distressed people with intellectual disabilities to manage their chaotic emotions. *Research and Practice in Intellectual and Developmental Disabilities, 10*, 1–15. https://doi.org/10.1080/23297018.2022.2106146

Deveau, R., & McGill, P. (2009). Physical interventions for adults with intellectual disabilities: Survey of use, policy, training and monitoring. *Journal of Applied Research in Intellectual Disabilities, 22*(2), 145–151. https://doi.org/10.1111/j.1468-3148.2008.00482.x

Emerson, E. (2001). *Challenging behaviour analysis and intervention in people with severe intellectual disabilities* (2nd ed.). Cambridge University Press.

Gore, N. J., Sapiets, S. J., Denne, L. D., Hastings, R. P., Toogood, S., MacDonald, A., Baker, P., Allen, D., Apanasionok, M. M., Austin, D., Bowring, D. L., Bradshaw, J., Corbett, A., Cooper, V., Deveau, R., Hughes, J. C., Jones, E., Lynch, M., McGill, P., et al. (2022). Positive Behavioural support in the UK: A state of the nation report. *International Journal of Positive Behavioural Support, 12*(1), 4–39.

Hayward, B. A., Poed, S., McKay-Brown, L., & McVilly, K. R. (2021). Introducing positive behaviour support (PBS) into disability services for successful adoption: A synthesised systematic review. *British Journal of Learning Disabilities, 49*(2), 145–161. https://doi.org/10.1111/bld.12363

Jones, E. (2013). Back to the future: Developing competent residential services for people with intellectual disabilities and challenging behaviour. *Advances in Mental Health and Intellectual Disabilities, 7*(1), 5–17. https://doi.org/10.1108/20441281311294657

Kim, R., & Dymond, S. K. (2020). What skills are critical for living in supported apartments and small group homes? *Journal of Developmental and Physical Disabilities, 32*(4), 665–681. https://doi.org/10.1007/s10882-019-09713-0

Langthorne, P., & McGill, P. (2012). An indirect examination of the function of problem behavior associated with fragile X syndrome and Smith-Magenis syndrome. *Journal of Autism and Developmental Disorders, 42*(2), 201–209. https://doi.org/10.1007/s10803-011-1229-6

Leif, E. S., Fox, R. A., Subban, P., & Sharma, U. (2023). 'Stakeholders are almost always resistant': Australian behaviour support practitioners' perceptions of the barriers and enablers to reducing restrictive practices. *International Journal of Developmental Disabilities, 69*(1), 66–82. https://doi.org/10.1080/20473869.2022.2116908

Lewis, N., Reynolds, E., Vale, M., Keenan, E., Hartland, A., Haines, M., & Davies, B. E. (2021). An evaluation of positive behavioural support implemented within an intensive community support service for people with learning disabilities who present with behaviours that challenge. *Journal of Intellectual Disabilities, 25*(3), 348–356. https://doi.org/10.1177/1744629519890962

McGill, P., Bradshaw, J., Smyth, G., Hurman, M., & Roy, A. (2020). Capable environments. *Tizard Learning Disability Review, 25*(3), 109–116. https://doi.org/10.1108/TLDR-05-2020-0007

McGill, P., Vanono, L., Clover, W., Smyth, E., Cooper, V., Hopkins, L., Barratt, N., Joyce, C., Henderson, K., Sekasi, S., Davis, S., & Deveau, R. (2018). Reducing challenging behaviour of adults with intellectual disabilities in supported accommodation: A cluster randomized controlled trial of setting-wide positive behaviour support. *Research in Developmental Disabilities, 81*, 143–154. https://doi.org/10.1016/j.ridd.2018.04.020

McGowan, S., McNally, K., & Vassos, M. (2017). The implementation of multicomponent positive behavioural interventions: Preliminary evidence of a negative relationship with challenging behaviour. *International Journal of Positive Behavioural Support, 7*(2), 3–12.

NDIS Quality and Safeguards Commission. (2020). Regulated restrictive practices guide.

NDIS Quality and Safeguards Commission. (2022). NDIS quality and safeguards commission activity report 1 April to 30 June 2022.

Ockenden, J., Ashman, B., & Beadle-Brown, J. (2014). Active support—fundamental to positive behaviour support. *Research and Practice in Intellectual and Developmental Disabilities, 1*(2), 98–107. https://doi.org/10.1080/23297018.2014.961528

Oliver, C., Woodcock, K. A., & Humphreys, G. W. (2009). The relationship between components of the Behavioural phenotype in Prader-Willi syndrome. *Journal of Applied Research in Intellectual Disabilities, 22*(4), 403–407. https://doi.org/10.1111/j.1468-3148.2008.00475.x

Olivier-Pijpers, V. C., Cramm, J. M., & Nieboer, A. P. (2020). Cross-sectional investigation of relationships between the organisational environment and challenging behaviours in support services for residents with intellectual disabilities. *Heliyon, 6*(8), e04751–e04751. https://doi.org/10.1016/j.heliyon.2020.e04751

Tournier, T., Heniks, A. H. C., Jahoda, A., Hastings, R. P., & Embregts, P. J. C. M. (2020). Developing a logic model for the triple-C intervention: A practice-derived intervention to support people with intellectual disability and challenging behavior. *Journal of Policy and Practice in Intellectual Disabilities, 17*(4), 297–307. https://doi.org/10.1111/jppi.12333

CHAPTER 10

Support Planning with People with Disabilities

Tal Araten-Bergman

Disability policy and practice focus on the human rights of people with disabilities, their quality of life and their exercise of choice and control. It places people with disabilities at the centre of decision-making about their lives, recognising their strengths, preferences and personal goals. Many countries have adopted person-centred approaches to service planning and delivery which individualise and organise service systems to maximise choice and control of the services and support received. Increasingly individualised funding mechanisms such as direct payments and personal budgets are used to allocate government funding directly to individuals so that they can purchase services based on their own desired outcomes and support needs.

Individualised funding and person-centred approaches require a significant change in the roles of all professionals involved in disability services and the way services are delivered and evaluated. Disability practice must shift away from professional assessments and judgements about the services a person needs to live a good life. Rather professionals and service

T. Araten-Bergman (✉)
Living with Disability Research Centre, La Trobe University,
Melbourne, VIC, Australia
e-mail: T.Araten-bergman@latrobe.edu.au

C. Bigby, A. Hough (eds.), *Disability Practice*,
https://doi.org/10.1007/978-981-99-6143-6_10

providers must strive for greater collaboration with the person with disability and others who know them well, to understand their support needs and preferences. Collaborative meetings of all the experts about a person's life including the person themselves and the people who know them in different ways and from different perspectives should lead to responses tailored to meet the unique needs and preferences of a person across different life domains.

The processes of *support planning* are fundamental to person-centred services and individualised funding. Through a collaborative process, support planning aims to identify what is most important to and for a person to live a good life, explore resources in their environment, and make decisions about the nature and quantity of services and supports needed to assist in having a good quality of life.

Support planning has become a primary task of the disability workforce. However, service providers, policymakers and people with disabilities themselves are often confused about the purpose and processes of support planning and what constitutes best practice. For example, research shows that planning is often mistaken for a short meeting with professional experts which aims to produce a static plan or planning is conceived to be a one-off meeting between the person, their significant others and a service provider. Such misunderstandings can mean key stakeholders underestimate the time, effort and skills necessary to effectively support people with disability to live the life they want (O'Brien & Lovett, 1993; Robertson et al., 2007; Taylor & Taylor, 2013).

This chapter aims to review the purposes of support planning, the different types of plans, the common principles and processes of good planning and to consider some of the complexities of putting these principles into practice to ensure plans are implemented and inform action. In the rest of the chapter, the term "professional" primarily refers to the service provider responsible for coordinating the planning processes and developing the support plan.

Support Needs and Support Planning

Contemporary disability practice has two basic assumptions. First is that people with disabilities have the same human needs as the general population (such as needs for information, health, housing, meaningful personal relationships, active engagement, choice and control). Second is that the quality of life and daily functioning of people with (and without) disabilities is significantly influenced by the availability of supports to meet their needs (Thompson et al., 2009; Thompson et al., 2002; van Loon et al., 2010).

Supports are defined as resources (such as skills, money, technologies and time) and services that aim to promote personal growth, interests, capabilities and opportunities for a person to function and live a good life (Thompson et al., 2002; Thompson et al., 2009). Supports can be provided by natural supporters (such as family, friends and community members), mainstream services (such as health, mental health education and justice), specialised services designed specifically for an individual (such as drop-in support) or specialised services designed for a specific group of service users with disability such as a social club, day centre or group home.

The need for supports is not unique to people with disabilities: everyone in their day-to-day life relies on a variety of supports and services (such as those provided by the education system, healthcare, housing and employment). However, for many people with disabilities, supports available from mainstream services are insufficient to realise the opportunities that life presents and they may require additional or different types of support to participate in society and to have a good quality of life. People with intellectual disabilities may need additional help to meet their needs; this help is often only available through specialist disability services, such as support to access and use mainstream services, or to make decisions or participate in their community.

Current disability practice aims to understand peoples' *support needs*. This means understanding how a person wants to live their life, what they want to do, what is and who are important to them, and what a person needs to stay safe and healthy. The depth and breadth of understanding sought about a person's support needs varies considerably depending on where support needs planning occurs. For example, it may only be superficial when the purpose of planning is the allocation of funding but may be very detailed and specific when the purpose of planning is to guide the direct provision of support to meet a person's aspirations to build social connections. It is widely acknowledged that every person's support needs are unique and reflect the gap between their characteristics and abilities, the available opportunities in their environment and how they want to live their life. Understanding a person's support needs, planning with them and providing the right type and amount of supports to them may bridge this gap and result in positive outcomes such as improved functioning, greater independence, better quality of life and social inclusion (Thompson et al., 2009).

Purpose and Key Principles of Support Planning

In the broadest sense, support planning is a systematic process where the person with disability, significant people in their life and professionals work collaboratively to identify what is most important to and for the person (their goals and support needs) and then develop strategies to utilise resources to enable the person to live the life they want. This open and collaborative exploratory process should result in a support plan—a document that outlines a person's goals and describes how these will be achieved through the involvement of people, services and resources (Sanderson, 2000).

An ideal plan explains clearly a person's desired outcomes and details specifically what will be done, when and by whom, thus setting a clear work plan for all people and services involved. Of course, many plans look very different from this ideal type. The level of detail they include about goals, needs, strategies and resources depends on where in the service system support planning occurs. Indeed, in service systems with individualised funding a person's initial support plan may simply deal with the allocation of funding. For example, in Australia's National Disability Insurance Scheme (NDIS), planners in the National Disability Insurance Agency (NDIA) develop high-level plans with scant details other than the volume of allocated funding. Such plans then cascade down and are progressively developed with greater levels of specificity by support coordinators, the person themselves or service providers.

Support planning is carried out by different organisations, such as federal government agencies that allocate funds (such as the NDIA), by support coordinators or case managers who aim to find and coordinate services to meet the support needs identified by funding agencies, or by staff in services contracted to deliver specific supports to a person.

Thus, plans take many shapes and forms depending on the context, the type of organisation where the planning is done and the desired outcome. Some plans may focus on a specific life domain or life course transition, and others on all domains and the whole of a person's life. For example, people with disability and their families might plan to address a particular life domain such as healthcare, education or leisure, or plan how to best support the person through certain life stages or transitions, such as starting or leaving school, or they may focus more comprehensively on a person's aspirations for their future lifestyle.

Regardless of the particular type of planning and its specific purpose and context, all planning processes should involve the person and others who are experts about aspects of their life. The key principles of planning processes are that it is: person centred, collaborative, individualised, focused on personal outcomes and dynamic,

- Person centred: planning processes focus on the person and how they want to live their life. The person is encouraged and supported to have as much choice and control over the planning process as possible and thus decisions about things that are important to them.
- Collaborative: planning processes are collaborative where people with disabilities, significant others who know them well and professionals share power and make decisions about support needs and services.
- Individualised: planning processes and plans reflect the unique circumstances of each person and their environment. All planning activities and decisions are tailored to the person's individual characteristics, values, life experience, age, gender, culture, heritage and language.
- Focused on personal outcomes: planning processes focus on understanding the person's goals, wishes and capabilities, articulating what specifically will contribute to their quality of life in the present and future and how to make it happen. Planning is not about fitting people into existing service models and solutions. Outcomes should be clear and measurable but also realistic and available.
- Dynamic: planning is a flexible, continuous, and dynamic process, designed to suit the person's changing circumstances, goals and priorities over time. Monitoring and review of a plan is an essential part of the process which results in ongoing listening, learning and future actions. Importantly, the planning process is not a one-off event.

Collaboration and shared power between the person themselves, professionals and service providers are key to good planning. While in the past people with disabilities were passive recipients of care and professionals were the experts, current practice requires that the person themselves and, where appropriate, those who care about them drive decision-making about support. Shifting power away from professionals does not detract from their roles as subject matter or system experts and reliance on their knowledge and expertise in working with people with disabilities, families and services and building partnerships to articulate needs and initiate actions. Support planning brings together people with disabilities as experts on their own life and professionals as "experts of the process". While all parties play an active role in planning processes, it is the responsibility of the professionals to build and sustain a collaborative approach and create a warm and safe environment to sustain effective processes.

Support planning processes are based on the notion that knowledge and understanding about support needs and effective solutions are created through an open and free dialogue. At the start of any planning process, neither the person nor the professional possesses all the knowledge required about needs and supports. Rather it is through purposeful engagement between the person, significant people in their lives and professionals that such knowledge is shared or created. This knowledge can then be used to reach informed decisions about desired goals and preferred supports necessary to formulate a plan. It is the professionals' role to create a safe space and to allow sufficient time for a free exchange of ideas and exploration of different options and solutions.

Many years of research in human service practice generally, and disability in particular, shows that a trusting relationship between professionals and service users results in more realistic and sustainable plans which then yield better outcomes for the person and more effective resource allocation for the service system (Collings et al., 2018; O'Brien & O'Brien, 2002).

Support Planning Processes

This section sets out the generic processes of planning, recognising that the exact nature of each step and the plan itself is heavily influenced by its purpose and context. If plans are to be successfully implemented, the planning process should explore as deeply as possible the person's situation, goals, support needs and strategies for meeting these. Good support planning addresses issues of capacity, functioning and health and safety. This requires a tailored process that includes:

1. Getting to know the person or pre-planning
2. Assessing support needs
3. Formulating the plan: setting goals, strategies and processes for monitoring and review

Support planning is a complex and iterative process, where the demarcation between each part is not always clear and which may involve moving backwards and forwards between different parts (Bigby & Frawley, 2010). Nevertheless, separating and describing each part of the process is useful for identifying the tasks and issues that each involves.

1. Getting to Know the Person or Pre-planning

The first part of the process is sometimes referred to as "pre-planning" and lays the foundation for the rest of the process. It is important for the professional to gain insight into how to communicate effectively with the person, who are the important people in the person's life and the support the person needs to be involved and to participate in the planning process. This requires the professional to spend time gathering and analysing information from a variety of sources about how the person communicates (e.g. verbally, using communication aids, how to tell if they are happy or not, comfortable or not with someone or something), how they learn and process information, how they make decisions and who supports them in making choices or expressing preferences. This information enables the professional to tailor the planning processes to be as beneficial as possible to the person (Collings et al., 2016; Dowse et al., 2016).

Getting to know the person involves more than reading or recording information: it is about spending time together building a trusting relationship and making sure that everyone involved understands their role, the purpose of the planning and how the support plan will be used. Too often pre-planning is undervalued and neglected or constrained by inadequate allocation of time and other resources.

2. Assessing Support Needs

This part of the process provides time and space to explore the person's goals and support needs in the context of their life. It seeks to garner evidence to inform decisions about desired outcomes and what support should be included in the plan to achieve these. It is important to understand that assessment is not a diagnostic process or an evaluation of whether the person is eligible for certain services (although exploring service options and issues of eligibility may be necessary as part of formulating a plan). Rather assessing support needs is about gathering and analysing information about the person, their environment, what is important *to* and *for* them to live a good life, and the supports required for them to maintain or improve their functioning and quality of life (Chenoweth, 2005; Rummery, 2002).

The scope and nature of information needed and the method of engaging in the assessment are determined by the purpose of planning and the mandate given to the professional. Nevertheless, even if a plan is focused on one area of a person's life such as employment, it may also require supports in other areas of their lives (such as transportation) to be considered. Effective assessment of support needs is a holistic and dynamic process that seeks to understand the various elements that impact the person's quality of life and functioning across multiple settings and environments.

The most vital information comes of course from the person themselves. Knowledge about the person, their situation, and their goals and needs can be gained through purposeful conversation and observation with the person across multiple settings over time. It is unlikely to be enough to simply ask a person what they want or need, as many people, particularly those with intellectual disabilities, find it difficult to conceptualise and articulate their needs. Moreover, many people lack the confidence, knowledge or experience to make informed choices about things they want for themselves (Priestley, 1998). Therefore, it is important for the professional as an "expert on the process" to support the person to think about different areas of their life, ask questions and raise new ideas, opportunities and possibilities (Milner & O'Byrne, 1998; Rummery, 2002). For example, the professional can ask questions such as the following: "How do you want to spend the day?" "What do you want to learn to do?" "Where do you want to live and with whom?" "Where do you want to work?" "Who do you want to spend time with?"

Particularly, when planning with people with intellectual disabilities, it is important to also include other sources of information. This may include, for example, perspectives of family and friends who know the person well or in different contexts and settings. It may also be helpful to interview service providers and review case notes and documents such as prior assessments, health checks and service reports.

Most organisations provide frameworks to guide the domains to be covered in the needs assessment or require a review of specific documents as evidence. While some require a broad exploratory process, others call for the use of standardised tools, such as the Supports Intensity Scales (SIS) (American Association on Intellectual and Developmental Disabilities 2015–2018) or the Inventory for Client and Agency Planning (ICAP)

(Bruininks et al., 1986) and the Instrument for the Classification and Assessment of Support Needs (I-CAN) (CDS, 2021).

Regardless of the specific format, for an assessment to be effective it must consider three overlapping factors: the person, their environment and the supports. This stage of the process seeks to gain:

An understanding of the *person*:

- Their current situation
- Their personal characteristics (including personality, cultural background, health and impairment)
- Their individual and family history and life circumstances (including developmental, social and cultural perspectives)
- Their social networks and current community participation patterns (social relationships, involvement in employment, leisure or voluntary activities)
- Their past experience using services, what has worked, what hasn't worked and why

An understanding of the *person's environment*:

- The opportunities and resources in their environment
- The accessibility and quality of these resources

An understanding of *supports:*

- The scope and function of supports and services being used by the person including mainstream, specialist and informal support
- Potential barriers and facilitators of supports

Next, it is important to gain insight into what is "important to" and "important for" the person. "Important to" the person is what matters to the person, their dreams and goals, and what it means for them to live a good life today and in the future (Sanderson, 2000). For example, where they would like to live and work, and what activities they want to participate in and with whom. Initially, in this part of the planning process, it is appropriate to support the person to explore their ideal vision, ensuring the discussion is not constrained by available resources or perceived barriers such as restricted funding or limitation in personal skills (O'Brien & O'Brien, 2002; O'Brien & Lovett, 1993). However, when engaged in the latter part of planning, making the best use of the available resources is clearly relevant.

In contrast, thinking about what is "important for" the person takes a more normative approach, focusing attention on what community standards might consider is necessary for a good life. For example, the plan could consider the person's need for participation in the community, taking on valued social roles, and staying healthy and safe in their environment (Sanderson, 2000).

Information gathering is not an end in itself. To be of value, the information gathered from different sources must be analysed and interpreted to help understand the person's goals, needs, risks and potential domains for change. This analysis provides the evidence on which decisions about goals, outcomes and potential strategies can be made. The assessment process also seeks to uncover and highlight potential challenges for implementation.

3. Formulating the Plan: Setting Goals, Strategies and Processes for Monitoring and Review

Support planning processes aim to formulate an optimistic but realistic support plan that sets out the person's prioritised outcomes and specifies strategies and actions that will lead to these (Thompson et al., 2017). As already discussed the scope, nature and format of a plan are determined by its purpose, context and the mandate given to the professional. Regardless of any particular format, every plan should include three elements:

1. Goal setting: what will the plan achieve? The person's goals and support needs phrased as valued outcomes: the things the person wants to achieve through the plan.
2. Identifying strategies: how goals are going to be met. Strategies to achieve goals, laying out specific activities and services to help the person meet their goals. This includes details about the types of support and services to be used, who will provide them, the amount required and who will fund them.
3. Monitoring and review processes. Processes for monitoring and review, which sets out how the plan will be implemented, managed and monitored, by whom and when, as well as when, by whom and under what circumstances the plan will be reviewed.

Goal Setting: What Will the Plan Achieve?

Goals represent what the person wants to achieve to live the life they want. Goals should be phrased as the desirable outcome the person wants and articulate what exactly will change in their life circumstances as a result of implementing the plan. Goals are personal and tailored specifically to each person's wants and needs, bringing together what is important to and for them in different life domains (see Chap. 2). The agreed set of goals should be phrased clearly and detailed in an observable and measurable way and set out a specific time frame for achievement.

A goal could be something that the person wants to do now or in the future, for example, participating in social and recreational activities: "In the next 12 months I want to go to the shopping centre by myself or with friends", or "I want to join a social club". A goal could be about relationships with others or social inclusion: "I want to have more friends", or "I want to go for family dinners". It could be something that the person wants to learn to do to build their capacity: "I want to be able to communicate more effectively with people", or "I want to cook my own meals". Or it could be something that would allow the person to be more independent and have more choice and control over their life: "I want to live in my own home", or "I want to travel independently".

Goals can be big or small, or short term or long term. Long-term goals usually involve complex changes that take time to achieve. Long-term goals often require more detailed planning, breaking big tasks into steps using short-term goals as stepping stones to larger goals.

Decisions about which goals are to be included in a plan require careful consideration and negotiation. The needs assessment process will have given an overall picture of the person and their vision for a good life but may have resulted in a long list of goals. It is unlikely that a support plan can efficiently include all the goals identified by the person or all areas of a person's life. Therefore, at this stage of the process, the discussion should focus on prioritising goals to be included in the plan.

The person's preferences should be the starting point for this discussion. As with the previous stage about envisioning a good life, it is important to remember that while some people are very clear about their goals, others may require help in identifying and articulating their priorities. It is the professional's role to help a person explore different elements in their life and to think about the changes that would most help them to live the life they want. Setting goals needs to be realistic to avoid failure and requires careful consideration of the resources required to meet them. Therefore, it is crucial at this stage to consider the person's capabilities as well as the availability of support services and resources in their environment.

Furthermore, sometimes the goals identified by the person are different from the needs seen by caregivers, families, friends and other professionals. For example, a person may aspire to participate in activities that may be seen by others as a risk to their health, safety and well-being or as unrealistic because of the person's skills and capacities. When these issues arise, it is the professional's role to support the person to articulate their needs and at the same time help family members voice their concerns. The professional helps the parties to balance the principle of dignity of risk with the duty of care. Then, the parties carefully work through their differences and reach a mutual agreement about goals and how the person can be best supported to reach them.

Negotiating goals requires open and genuine discussion about practical possibilities and constraints. A good planning process seeks to balance the person's choice and what is realistic in a given context. For example, Mary's goal is to "have a job and earn my own money", but the needs assessment and family members recognise that she struggles to wake up in the morning on time. It is the professional's role to lead an honest discussion about what it may take for Mary to find a job and reflect on how important it may be to improve her time management. If Mary agrees the importance of this and is willing to work towards it, the plan could include Mary's long-term goals as "getting a job" broken into shorter-term goals such as "in the next 12 months I want to be able to manage my time better so I can be ready on time to go to my morning activities".

Identifying Strategies: How Goals Are Going to Be Met

This part of the plan is closely aligned with the goals and is about the "how". It sets out what services, supports and particular steps are required to achieve the person's goals. Each goal usually has several strategies detailing the activities, services and supports (what would happen), responsibilities (who will do it) and time frame (when would this happen, for how long).

When considering strategies, it is important to explore potential formal and informal sources of support that may assist the person in achieving their goals. These could include:

- The person's skills, knowledge and strengths—what can they do by themself or with support
- The person's informal network, including family, friends, neighbours and volunteers
- Existing and available paid support (disability-specific and mainstream services)
- Existing and available technologies and possible environmental modification
- Existing and available funding mechanisms

As with all other parts of the planning process, identifying strategies is a collaborative effort: the person, the professional and others the person wants to be involved in their life should be invited to contribute their expertise and knowledge in identifying ways to accomplish the person's goals. The decision about what strategies to include must reflect the person's preferences and the availability and accessibility of support and services (Bigby & Frawley, 2010). There are many different possible ways of reaching a goal. It is important to consider what might be the most effective pathway for the person at this point in time. For example, if Jim's goal is "I want to learn how to cook my own meals", strategies could be:

- The NDIS will fund $300 to purchase some adaptive equipment such as a switch for the blender and a tipping kettle; Jim and his mother will liaise with the Independent Living Centre to explore available technology by the end of October.
- Two hours of support every weekday (10 hours a week) will help Jim to cook lunch and dinner—the support coordinator will organise this with the local disability support service by November 14.

When describing the strategies, it is important to use clear, specific and objective language. Where possible, avoid ambiguity or the possibility of misinterpretation by giving measurable milestones or actions. For example, it's better to say 'twice a week' than "regularly".

This stage also requires the professional to facilitate an in-depth discussion about potential barriers to supports and how they will be addressed in the plan. This might involve considering the person's motivation, past experiences and availability of resources and funding. This will ensure that any barriers stemming from limited funding and the availability of formal and informal supports and services are clearly recognised, addressed and resolved before the plan is implemented.

Monitoring and Review Processes

Planning processes must include discussion about the management of the plan, monitoring and review. The professional leading the preparation of the plan may not be the person responsible for its implementation and tasks such as finding and coordinating services or day-to-day plan management. This makes it crucial to identify who takes responsibility for organising and implementing strategies for every goal and who will have overall responsibility for coordinating strategies and monitoring progress.

Planning is an ongoing process; personal preferences, resource availability and social environments change over time. Reviewing the plan and evaluating its outcomes help to ensure that all actions, strategies and supports are revised if they are not effective or no longer meet the person's needs and goals.

Conclusion

Support planning is a core component of policy and service provision for people with disabilities and their families. Supporting people to develop a plan is now a primary task of the disability workforce. In this chapter, we identified the core principles and processes of successful support planning.

It is important to remember that plans are merely means to an end and are meaningful only when they are implemented effectively and result in a better quality of life and choice and control for the person. Successful support planning requires professionals to build partnerships with the person and the important people in their life and services, to guide an open and genuine exploration of the person's needs and goals, and to reach an agreement about how to meet them. This requires considering different perspectives about the person's situation, resolving tensions, identifying priorities, negotiating resources and considering opportunities for change. It is only through this shared understanding that meaningful goals can be identified and prioritised, and realistic strategies can be planned and implemented.

Take Home Messages

- Disability policy aims to enable people with disability to have a good quality of life and to exercise choice and control over the services and supports they receive.
- Support planning aims to develop a shared understanding of a person's support needs in the context of their life and identify the supports a person requires to live the life they want.
- Support planning has various purposes, for example, determining funding, setting broad life goals and creating detailed blueprints for the delivery of specific supports.
- Support planning is carried out by staff with differing roles and in a wide range of organisations: for example, central government agencies which allocate funding packages for support; support coordinators and case managers add more detail about needs and goals to funding plans and find and coordinate services to meet these; and staff in services contracted to deliver specific supports to a person who must plan for how these will be delivered.
- Regardless of differences, processes of support planning are based on principles of being person centred, collaborative, individualised, focused on personal outcomes and dynamic.
- Support planning has three core processes: getting to know the person or pre-planning, assessing support needs and formulating the plan.

References

American Association on Intellectual and Developmental Disabilities (2015-2018). *Supports intensity scales.* AAIDD.

Bigby, C., & Frawley, P. (2010). *Social work and intellectual disability: Working for change.* London: Palgrave MacMillan.

Bruininks, R. H., Hill, B. K., Weatherman, R. F., & Woodcock, R. W. (1986). *Inventory for client and agency planning.* Riverside Publishing.

CDS. (2021). *Instrument for the classification and assessment of support needs (version 6).* Centre for Disability Studies University of Sydney.

Chenoweth, L. (2005). *The road to social work & human service practice: An introductory text.* Thomson Learning.

Collings, S., Dew, A., & Dowse, L. (2016). Support planning with people with intellectual disability and complex support needs in the Australian National

Disability Insurance Scheme. *Journal of Intellectual and Developmental Disability, 41*(3), 272–276. https://doi.org/10.3109/13668250.2016.1151864
Collings, S., Dew, A., & Dowse, L. (2018). Unpacking the complexity of planning with persons with cognitive disability and complex support needs. *Journal of Applied Research in Intellectual Disabilities, 31*(1), 142–151. https://doi.org/10.1111/jar.12381
Dowse, L., Wiese, M., Dew, A., Smith, L., Collings, S., & Didi, A. (2016). More, better, or different? NDIS workforce planning for people with intellectual disability and complex support needs. *Journal of Intellectual and Developmental Disability, 41*(1), 81–84. https://doi.org/10.3109/13668250.2015.1125868
Milner, J., & O'Byrne, P. (1998). *Assessment in social work*. Palgrave.
O'Brien, J., & Lovett, H. (1993). *Finding a Way Toward Everyday Lives: The Contribution of Person-Centered Planning*. Pennsylvania Office of Mental Retardation.
O'Brien C., & O'Brien, J. (2002). The origins of person-centered planning. In P. Vietze & S. Holburn (Eds.), *Person-centered planning: Research, practice, and future directions*. Baltimore.
Priestley, M. (1998). Constructions and creations: Idealism, materialism and disability theory. *Disability and Society, 13*(1), 75–94. https://doi.org/10.1080/09687599826920
Robertson, J., Emerson, E., Hatton, C., Elliott, J., McIntosh, B., Swift, P., Krinjen-Kemp, E., Towers, C., Romeo, R., Knapp, M., Sanderson, H., Routledge, M., Oakes, P., & Joyce, T. (2007). Person-centred planning: Factors associated with successful outcomes for people with intellectual disabilities. *Journal of Intellectual Disability Research, 51*(3), 232–243. https://doi.org/10.1111/j.1365-2788.2006.00864.x
Rummery, K. (2002). *Disability, citizenship and community care: A case for welfare rights?* Ashgate.
Sanderson, H. (2000). *Person-centred planning: Key features and approaches*. York.
Taylor, J. E., & Taylor, J. A. (2013). Person-centered planning: Evidence-based practice, challenges, and potential for the 21st century. *Journal of Social Work in Disability & Rehabilitation, 12*(3), 213–235. https://doi.org/10.1080/1536710X.2013.810102
Thompson, J. R., Bradley, V. J., Buntinx, W. H. E., Schalock, R. L., Shogren, K. A., Snell, M. E., Wehmeyer, M. L., Borthwick-Duffy, S., Coulter, D. L., Craig, E. M., Gomez, S. C., Lachapelle, Y., Luckasson, R. A., Reeve, A., Spreat, S., Tassé, M. J., Verdugo, M. A., & Yeager, M. H. (2009). Conceptualizing supports and the support needs of people with intellectual disability. *Intellectual and Developmental Disabilities, 47*(2), 135–146. https://doi.org/10.1352/1934-9556-47.2.135

Thompson, J. R., Hughes, C., Schalock, R. L., Silverman, W., Tassé, M. J., Bryant, B., Craig, E. M., & Campbell, E. M. (2002). Integrating supports in assessment and planning. *Mental Retardation, 40*(5), 390–405.

Thompson, J. R., Wehmeyer, M. L., Shogren, K. A., & Seo, H. (2017). The supports paradigm and intellectual and developmental disabilities. In K. A. Shogren, M. L. Wehmeyer, & N. N. Singh (Eds.), *Handbook of positive psychology in intellectual and developmental disabilities translating research into practice*. Springer International Publishing: Imprint: Springer.

van Loon, J., Claes, C., Vandevelde, S., Van Hove, G., & Schalock, R. L. (2010). Assessing individual support needs to enhance personal outcomes. *Exceptionality: The Official Journal of the Division for Research of the Council for Exceptional Children, 18*(4), 193–202. https://doi.org/10.1080/09362835.2010.513924

CHAPTER 11

The Right to Participate in Decision Making: Supported Decision Making in Practice

Christine Bigby

Most people do not notice the decisions they make throughout every day which determine what their day will be like. For example, what time to get up, what to wear, whether to turn the radio on, whether to exercise before or after breakfast or whether to have the day off. Too often decision making only becomes visible when 'big decisions' need to be made—where to go on holiday, whether to apply for a new job, whether to move house. This might be when people stop to think about the processes involved in decision making and why these are important. All the decisions a person makes, whether little or big, influence their life in some way, and contribute to their sense of autonomy and self-determination: the choice and control a person has over their life. Yet too often people with disabilities are denied the right to make decisions and others make decisions for them. This may occur informally, through the everyday actions of supporters—be they staff or family members—or formally when supporters have a specific mandate, having been appointed as a person's nominee or guardian. Denying the right of people with disabilities to make decisions happens for

C. Bigby (✉)
Living with Disability Research Centre, La Trobe University, Melbourne, VIC, Australia
e-mail: C.Bigby@latrobe.edu.au

C. Bigby, A. Hough (eds.), *Disability Practice*,
https://doi.org/10.1007/978-981-99-6143-6_11

many reasons: fear of risks, paternalistic attitudes that people are incapable of understanding the options or of knowing what is best for themselves, rigid service systems organised around managerial needs or staff preferences—think for a moment about rosters and working hours—or simply a lack of supporter's time or skills to provide good support for decision making.

This chapter considers the significance of decision making to the lives of people with disabilities and changing expectations about their rights to participate in decision making since the 2006 United Nations Convention on the Rights of Persons with Disabilities. The chapter explains the processes and describes the skills required for the practice of good decision support with people with disabilities, through making decision making visible and the need for support explicit.

Why Decision Making Is Significant

The right to make decisions about one's own life and be involved in collective decisions about civic and political issues that impact on communities through, for example, casting a vote or participating in an advisory group are important features of citizenship and human rights (United Nations, 2006). Choice and control by people with disabilities is a core theme of contemporary disability policy. It is realised through individuals making decisions about things such as their personal goals, preferred supports and types of services. Indeed, the shift to individualised funding through schemes such as Australia's National Disability Insurance Scheme (NDIS) relies on a marketplace of services and people with disabilities being consumers and making decisions about which services to purchase. In this way not only do individuals control what services they receive, but as part of the bigger consumer group their decisions help to shape the type of services or organisations that thrive and those that don't. In theory at least, decisions by consumers in market systems drive up service quality and determine what is produced (Considine, 2022).

Making decisions is important for psychological and social wellbeing. It improves self-confidence, and by increasing a person's sense of mastery over their environment helps in developing skills and a sense of self. In the excerpt below, a parent of a young man with intellectual disability talks about the impact on her son when she tried to give him more support to make his own decisions.

> He's making more and more decisions himself. Like, smaller ones but he's taking ownership of them a little bit more. So, in terms of what he wants to eat, where he wants to eat sometimes if we're not eating at home, what he wants to wear. ... He just beams. He's a different person. There's a smile on his face. His shoulders are upright and it's like, 'I'm choosing this and I'm making it happen. I'm not waiting for someone else to lead me'. (Bigby et al., 2022, p. 6362)

This isn't only relevant to people with mild intellectual disabilities, as the comments from a parent of a women with severe intellectual disabilities illustrate. He describes the noticeable changes to his daughter's communication and self-determination as he tried to pay more attention to interpreting her preferences.

> ...a little bit of increase, the way that she communicates things...she has become more stubborn if she doesn't want to go somewhere. Like if it's time to leave the house and she's not ready or doesn't want to go, it's actually become more difficult to convince her to go to the front door. (Bigby et al., 2022, p. 6362)

In contrast, it can be belittling and hurtful when supporters fail to respect a person's preferences or simply take over their decisions. In this excerpt, a self-advocate explains what this feels like for him.

> There have been times that supporters have treated me like a child, telling us what to do, not as an independent person. We can feel like we're looked down upon a bit. ... When you're an adult, you want to be able to be independent and do what you want, but as well as ... being treated fairly with whatever decision you want to do in a very respectful fashion (Bigby et al., 2023, p. 32 and unpublished data).

Respecting the rights of people to make decisions for themselves also sends powerful messages that help to counter paternalistic public attitudes. There is a sense too that the intentional processes of supporting people with disabilities to make their own decisions act as a safeguard against abuse or exploitation, through putting in place principles that guide practice and the chances of more than one person being involved in decision support. As self-advocates say about support for decision making:

> If everyone's listening to me, then I'm much likely to be living the life that I want to live and be free of those abuses. (Bigby et al., 2023, p. 384)

> If you have the right supports, you can gain confidence – you do something with support such as catching a bus and you end up having the confidence to do it on your own. (Bigby et al., 2023, p. 31)

Taking Away Rights to Decision Making

Despite personal and wider social benefits of making one's own decisions, a significant body of research suggests that people with intellectual disabilities or other forms of cognitive impairment are denied the right to make decisions (Bigby et al., 2015). This ranges from day to day decisions at home or the community, where a support worker's preferences may swamp those of the person they are supporting, to less frequent decisions about goals, planning for services, purchases or health related issues. For example, two studies about NDIS planning found that all but one of the participants with mild intellectual disabilities reported that a family member had largely determined what was in their plan and overridden, failed to listen or silenced their own perspective (Bigby, 2020, p. 7). This is indicative of the failure of systems such as the NDIS to translate policy into practice. It is not sufficient, as the NDIS legislation does, to assert that all people with disabilities can make decisions. Rather systems must embed expectations around support for decision making into their operations and ensure there are processes for at least scrutinising how supporters arrive at their interpretation of a person's preferences.

Supporters may take over decision making in the moment—by neglecting to consult a person about their preferences or overriding them—or supporters may subtly try to influence a person's decisions. Subtle influences include, for example, limiting the options they support a person to consider—'you can have salad or vegetables with dinner'—or by framing some options more favourably than others—'wouldn't you prefer to go a new sports centre rather than the usual one where you are not likely to meet any new people'.

Decision making rights may be formally removed from a person with disability through the appointment of another person to make decisions for them. That person is known as a *substitute decision maker* and may be given the power to make decisions they consider to be in the 'best interests' of the person. Appointment of substitute decision makers goes as far back as the Middle Ages, although their powers, the terminology and mechanisms used have evolved over time and differ between countries. Examples of mechanisms for appointment of substitute decision makers for people with disability in Australia include the nominee provisions of Centrelink and the NDIS, the variously named tribunals in each State and Territory with power to appoint guardians and financial administrators, and State and Territory legislation to appoint 'persons responsible' for health related decisions if a person is deemed not to have capacity to make a decision for themselves (Bigby et al., 2023). Appointments such as these reflect a way of thinking about decision making that is contrary to universal human rights and assert a person must have *capacity* to make their own decisions; that is, they must understand the decision, the available options, the implications of their preferences and the potential risks of harm these may entail.

Notably, since the introduction of the NDIS a whole new class of nominees has arisen and the number of guardians appointed for people with intellectual disabilities has increased substantially. These are perhaps unintended consequences of the NDIS Act which embraces the presumption of capacity (National Disability Insurance Scheme Act 2013, s. 17A (1)). But this may also be due to the increased opportunities the scheme presents for decision making, coupled with the necessity for people with disabilities to enter into individual contracts as customers of disability services and uncertainty about the legal standing of some people to do this.

The Right to Support with Decision Making

The Convention on the Rights of Persons with Disabilities (CRPD) and, more recently, in Australia critiques of the NDIS have heightened the need for new ways of thinking about decision making by people with disabilities and reform of laws and policy. Article 12 of the CRPD articulates rights to autonomy and self-determination by recognising the right of people with disabilities to 'enjoy legal capacity on an equal basis with others' and requires State parties to 'take appropriate measures to provide access by persons with disabilities to the support they may require in exercising their legal capacity' (United Nations, 2006, Article 12 (2)–(3)).

Although Article 12 is framed in a somewhat legalistic manner, subsequent work on its meaning calls for the abolition of all forms of substitute decision making (United Nations Committee on the Rights of Persons with Disabilities, 2014). In its place the concept of supported decision making is promoted as a framework for upholding the decision making rights of people with disabilities. Supported decision making rests on four principles similar to those proposed in 2014 report by the Australian Law Reform Commission:

Principle 1: The equal right to make decisions All adults have an equal right to make decisions that affect their lives and to have those decisions respected.

Principle 2: Support All people who require support in decision-making must be provided with access to the support necessary for them to make, communicate and participate in decisions that affect their lives.

Principle 3: Will, preferences and rights The will, preferences and rights of people who may require decision-making support must direct decisions that affect their lives.

Principle 4: Safeguards Laws, legal and policy frameworks must contain appropriate and effective safeguards in relation to interventions for people who may require decision-making support, including to prevent abuse and undue influence (Australian Law Reform Commission, 2014, p. 11).

In essence these principles assert that people with disabilities have the right to make decisions about their lives, to have the support they need to ensure that all decisions reflect their short term preferences and the longer term values that direct their lives. Further, the principles assert that people with disabilities are protected from the influence or conflicts of interests of supporters.

The abolition of any form of substitute decision making, together with the application of these principles of supported decision making in the real world, raises some very difficult issues. For example:

- How do the principles apply to the situation of people with profound intellectual disabilities who are not able to participate directly in decision making no matter how skilled the supporter and whose preferences will have to be interpreted by supporters?
- How to reconcile competing rights of people with disabilities—the right to be safe and the right to make decisions?
- What is society's tolerance for the risk of serious harm to a person with disability that may result from their right to make a decision?

- What safeguards will be effective but do not remove the right of a person to make decisions?
- How can the trustworthiness and neutrality of supporters be ensured?

These difficulties help to understand why the principles of supported decision making have not been fully incorporated in law in Australia or elsewhere, and why supported decision making remains an uncertain and contested concept.

Recent Australian research for the Royal Commission into Violence, Abuse, Neglect and Exploitation of People with Disability (2022) suggests a way of thinking about supported decision making that tackles some of these difficult questions. It does this by moving away from a binary between substitute decision making being 'bad' and supported decision making being 'good'. Rather it proposes that the will and preferences of a person with disability should take precedence in all decision making situations whoever is making the actual decision. Table 11.1 captures this approach.

The principled approach to supported decision making is reflected in legal reforms to guardianship in some Australian states, such as Victoria, which require a substitute decision maker to find out a person's will and preferences, act in accordance with them and only override them to prevent serious harm (Guardian and Administration Act 2019, Victoria).

Service providers must understand the legal context they work in, as it limits their powers to interfere with a person's decision making. In particular, it guides support by setting out what they must do if they are concerned about serious risk of harm to a person or there is uncertainty or conflict among supporters. Importantly, good support for decision making does not have to wait for legal or policy reform. For people with cognitive disabilities who use services, most decision support occurs as part of the everyday practice of staff. Outside of the legal sphere, supported decision making is becoming a commonly used term, referring to the:

> ...everyday, practical process of support whereby an individual has a supporter who assists the individual to make decisions by collecting information, providing explanations, and helping the individual to have their decision-making autonomy respected. (Then et al., 2018, p. 64)

When supported decision making is understood in this way, it can be used by anyone anywhere in disability or mainstream services systems.

Table 11.1 Towards a principled approach to supported decision making

Binary approach	*Principled approach*
EITHER supported decision-making: The person retains control of their decision, actively participates in making it and is supported to do so. The person is supported to make decisions that reflect their will and preferences. Decisions are based on a person's stated will and preferences, not supporters' 'best interpretation' of will and preferences. **OR substitute decision making:** If a person is deemed lacking capacity to make a decision and communicate their will and preferences, then supported decision making no longer applies and substitute decision making becomes necessary based on the person's 'best interests'.	**A CONTINUUM of decision making supports (including some forms of substitution)** The person is supported to maximise their autonomy in making decisions. Decisions are based on a person's stated will and preferences. Where a person cannot communicate their will and preferences, supporters' best interpretation of the person's will and preferences is applied ('will and preferences substitute decision-making'). The dignity and importance of taking risk is acknowledged and supported. In very limited circumstances, where a person's stated or inferred will and preferences involve risk of serious, imminent physical or financial harm with lasting consequences to themselves (including incurring civil or criminal liability), and that person is unable to understand that risk even with support, a substitute decision can be made as a last resort with the person's personal and social wellbeing being, as well as will and preferences, guiding decision making ('personal and social wellbeing substitute decision-making').

Source Bigby et al., (2023).

Direct support workers or support coordinators may directly support a person to make decisions; managers may ensure their staff have adequate training in supported decision making and that organisational policies require the use of supported decision making. Alternatively, advocates or family members may ask about how supporters are providing decision support by getting them to describe the processes they have used.

Evidence Informed Supported Decision Making

People with disabilities can be involved in many different types of decisions when supporters provide the right opportunities and support. Decision making is characterised by diversity; every decision is different and the support a person needs to make each decision will be different. The support needed depends on the decision and its context, the person and their skills and knowledge about the decision and options available, their preferences about the options, the constraints on the options, the risks involved, and the perspectives and skills of the supporters involved and those of other people who may be affected by the decision. For example, a decision about going on holiday will be affected by the person's:

- Context: Will they need support to go on holiday, and will it have to fit into their existing schedule of support from service providers?
- Knowledge of the available options: Do they have experience of the different places they might go or places they might stay?
- Preferences about where to go, what to do, how to get there, and when to go: What do they like doing. Do they like the sea, nature, walking or sailing? Do they prefer driving or going on a train or flying?
- Constraints: How much money do they have to spend on a holiday?
- Other people impacted by the decision: For example, what are the preferences of their friend who is coming along too?

Providing good support for decision making takes time; it relies on knowing a person well, understanding their support needs, their social and service contexts, an attitude that the person is capable of participating in decision making and does have preferences, and a commitment to creating opportunities for decision making. Supporting decision making may happen quickly and many times during a day as part of good Active Support practice (see Chap. 7) or may require dedicated time over several weeks. Self-advocates and service providers describe what good decision support looked like in the following ways:

> Three people in my house can't use an iPad or phone – so need to have a worker who 'notices things in that person, notices little things that they enjoy...' or activities they do. Two of them have parents involved but they can't speak to let their parents know they're not being supported to make decisions. Sometimes you just need to observe, take the time. (Self–advocate)

> ... it was extra time and questioning me in all different ways to make sure I understood it. (Self-advocate)

> It takes time ultimately to provide supported decision making to an individual. It is based on trust and relationship, so even if you have the skills and go into supported decision making as a profession, with tools for communication support and getting to know the person it takes time (Service provider). (Bigby et al., 2023, p. 80)

The La Trobe Support for Decision Making Practice Framework

The La Trobe Support for Decision Making Practice Framework (The Framework) is an evidence informed framework for supported decision making. Designed for supporters, it describes the principles of practice, the steps involved in decision support, and the range of strategies that can be used. When staff or families are trained to use The Framework and it is built into organisational expectations, they are more likely to provide support aligned with human rights and the principles of supported decision making (Bigby, Douglas, & Smith, 2022; Bigby, Douglas, et al., 2022a; Douglas et al., 2020). As well as a guide for supporters, The Framework acts as a checklist that can be used to hold supporters to account by describing the processes they have used (Fig. 11.1).

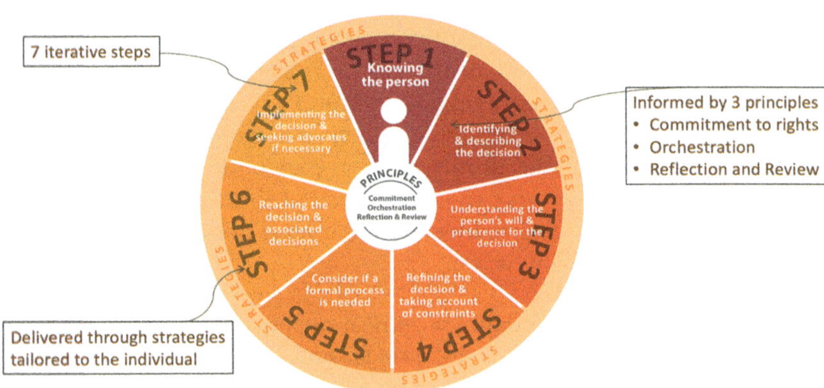

Fig. 11.1 La Trobe Support for Decision Making Practice Framework

The Framework has seven iterative steps and three principles and is delivered through a range of strategies tailored to each individual. The seven steps are common to all decision making support but don't always happen in the same order: a supporter may move backwards and forwards between the steps.

Step 1. Knowing the Person

Knowing the person is fundamental to person centred and individualised decision support and enables supporters to select the best strategies for each step of the process, such as how to adjust their communication or to scaffold information (that is, structuring the way in which information is shared in order to make understanding easier). Knowing a person requires information about things such as their personality, strengths, weaknesses, skills, likes, dislikes, social connections, aspirations for the future and short term preferences. It can be pieced together from the person themselves and other sources; family members may know about a person's history, a GP about their health, service providers about their supports and professionals about formal assessments of communication or functional abilities. Whoever is leading the decision support processes should complement information from other sources with their own observations and experiences with the person to build a rich picture about the person.

This step is challenging for paid supporters who come into a person's life for a specific decision or who are allocated only a little time to get to know them. It may be particularly difficult if you are working with a person with severe intellectual disabilities who cannot tell you about themselves. Supporters need to find and take time to read existing information such as support plans, seek out others who know the person, and spend time with the person as they move through different parts of their daily life. Generic skills such as active listening, observation, giving time to respond, adapting communication, as well as adopting a curious stance are all useful for this step.

Step 2. Identifying and Describing the Decision

This step helps to ensure decision support starts from the beginning, and that other decisions have not already been made without the person. For example, if a supporter identifies the decision as what type of home to move to, they might query when and how a decision to move at all was made. This step helps in being clear about the timing and scope of the decision, when it has to be made, if it is urgent, who else or what formal systems or services should be involved, the potential consequences for the person or others and other associated decisions that might need to be made. For example, a paid decision supporter spent several meetings with a middle aged man with intellectual disability who had sought help in making decisions about using his NDIS funding. The first thing she did was go through each of the goals in the plan with him to prioritise them. They decided that the goal of continuing to work on his anxiety and self-confidence was the most important to him. By knowing about the services the man was already using, the supporter identified the decision as being about finding a good psychologist and whether he should use his NDIS funds to continue to see the psychologist he had seen previously (but who could no longer be funded by the health system) or find a new one.

Step 3. Understanding the Person's Will and Preferences for the Decision

This step involves 'blue sky thinking', in which supporters assist the person to explore all the possible options, understand the implications of each, and think about which they prefer. This step may be as straightforward as identifying options and discussing the pros and cons of each. For example, helping a person to think about the different types of fitness classes they could attend, by listing their previous classes, talking about their experiences of each and then ranking them from best to worst.

Just talking through options may not be a good strategy. A person may not have experienced many of the possible options and find it hard to imagine what they are like and thus what their preferences are. One strategy is assisting the person to try out options and observe their reactions. Similarly, it may also be important for a person to experience the potentially negative consequences of their preferences. Here a risk enabling approach is useful. This involves trying out a risky option but also minimising any potential harm (Bigby, Douglas, & Hamilton, 2018). For example, as part of deciding about travelling independently, a travel trainer might shadow a person as they travel to identify difficulties they encounter and step in if necessary or prepare a help card for a person to give to a stranger.

It is important to take time, listen carefully and explore all the possible options. Supporters must take care not to influence the person in this step by, for example, disclosing their own preferences, filtering out options they don't like or don't think are possible, presenting options in biased ways or persuading the person towards those they prefer. Supporters should avoid focussing too much on risks and practicalities, or on making the 'right decision' for a person's wellbeing. A common mistake is to consider the constraints on a decision (Step 4) before exploring all the options (Step 3). This unnecessarily restricts options and means risky or impractical preferences are ignored. Allowing sufficient time to consider options at Step 3 provides the basis for prioritising preferences and understanding constraints at Step 4.

Step 4. Refining the Decision and Taking Account of Constraints

In this step, supporters assist the person to prioritise the options they prefer and take account of constraints without compromising their preferred decision. A decision is a choice that can be acted upon, either by the person themselves, supporters or advocates. Decisions are constrained by many things, and preferences must often be refined to take account of them. Constraints are things like money, time or support, the impact on others, attitudes of others, organisational policies or risks to safety or longer term wellbeing. For example, refining preferences to take account of money may mean helping the person select a purchase within their budget or postpone it until they have sufficient funds. Risk of potential harm is a common constraint and strategies for enabling risk can be suggested, such as equipping a person to be confident to seek help if they get lost on public transport. But rather than helping someone to experience consequences of risky options to help determine their preferences, the aim of enabling risk at this step is to help find ways of carrying through preferences into decisions by minimising any potential harm.

Thinking about a person's *will* as well as preferences is useful at this step, especially if constraints seem insurmountable. A person's will is the long term vision for their life, such as wanting to be healthy or independent, whereas preferences are immediate wishes or desires (Szmukler, 2019). A person's preferred option for a decision about travelling more independently may be to learn to drive. This may be so constrained by their poor literacy skills that it is practically unrealisable. A supporter might assist the person to refine their preference for learning to drive to one that helps them to stay true to their will of being independent but is more practical, such as learning to use the Uber app.

This step highlights how easily supporters can undermine rights to self-determination by emphasising constraints and suggesting alternatives to a person's preferences. It also requires supporters to consider whether they should take action to override a decision if the constraints on a preferred decision are significant or the risks to a person's safety great. In considering this, supporters rely on their understanding of a person's will and exploration of alternatives that are as close as possible to their preferences. As the next step suggests, such actions must be deeply considered and may require use of a formal processes.

Step 5. Consider if a Formal Process Is Needed

This step is influenced by context, and the role and standing of supporters. Most decision support is informal; that is, supporters have no formal legal standing in respect of the person's decision making. The judgements of decision supporters are guided by their knowledge about disability policy, their own principles or the policies of their employer, and are reliant on their skills and support they get from supervisors or peers. There may be situations that a supporter cannot resolve: when they judge a person's preferences may result in significant harm, when there is conflict among those involved in the decision or one of the supporters wants to override a person's preferences. Conflict arises when others question whether a person's preferences are realistic, accurately reflect their desires or are the result of undue influence or coercion. Many studies, for example, find conflict between accommodation support staff and family members of a person with disability about things such as holiday destinations, meals and dress codes (Bigby, Douglas, et al., 2022b; Bigby et al., 2019).

In many circumstances, where there is no immediate danger, it is preferable for supporters to seek out a process for mediation or appointing a guardian, rather than overriding preferences or leaving conflict unresolved (which often also leads to preferences being disregarded). Using formal processes can mean there are greater safeguards for the person's rights. Deciding if a formal process is necessary and taking action towards it should include the person themselves as much as possible, and in some situations finding them an independent advocate. The relevant State or Territory legislation and policies of disability support organisations will determine the available options and the steps supporters need to take to instigate a formal process. If a substitute decision maker is appointed, the knowledge of informal supporters will be important in helping to inform the decision making process of the substitute decision maker, remembering that substitute decision makers are increasingly required to make decisions based on the person's will and preferences unless there is a serious risk of harm to the person or others from doing so.

Step 6. Reaching the Decision and Associated Decisions

In this step a decision is made that reflects the person's prioritised preferences as closely as possible. In some instances, a decision may be formally recorded and communicated to someone else such as a support coordinator or advocate, who will be responsible for getting it implemented. It is also important to assist the person to think about the consequences of their decision, its likely implications for other parts of their life and the other decisions that may now need to be made. Decisions are like Russian Babushka dolls: they sit within each other, and as one decision is made another may appear. In supporting a person to think about associated decisions, the iterative nature of decision support practice is clear as you loop back to Step 2, by identifying and describing other decisions.

Step 7. Implementing the Decision and Seeking Advocates if Necessary

Acting on a decision is often the responsibility of other people in a person's life rather than the decision supporter. There are dangers that decisions will not be acted upon if they are not seen by others as important or they don't agree with them (Burgen, 2016). In such cases an advocate may be needed to ensure a decision is taken seriously and to oversee its implementation. This step helps to illustrate differences between the role of advocates and decision supporters. Advocates often work with a person to get a decision that has already been made to be implemented and decision supporters support the person to participate in making the decision.

Principles of Decision Support Practice

The Framework also has three principles that underpin all aspects of decision support practice. These include Commitment, Orchestration, and Reflection and Review:

1. *Commitment* to the person and their rights. This principle means supporters have a relationship with the person they support based on equity and respect for their rights. An explicit commitment to a person's rights helps supporters to avoid inadvertently using the so called 'best interest test' as the touchstone for support.
2. *Orchestration*. This principle points to the shared nature of decision support practice. That means bringing in others involved in the person's life or who have expertise about the decision at hand. It is based on there being a supporter who leads the process and who draws in and coordinates other paid or unpaid supporters and mediates any differences between them.
3. *Reflection and Review*. This principle emphasises self-awareness and continuous reflection on practice. Being self-reflective through all steps helps supporters to be conscious of their own influence, values or stake in the decision and better maintain a neutral approach that puts these aside.

The Framework is the basis for a simple checklist to help supporters review and describe their actions at each step of the process, reflecting on the principle and strategies they have used. The free online training resources developed as part of The Framework include this checklist and other tools that can be downloaded (Bigby et al., 2019).

Strategies

Supporters draw on many strategies as they move through The Framework's steps and apply the principles to their practice. These must be tailored for each individual, and specific to each decision and context. Some strategies have been described in earlier sections, and may include

- Adjusting communication
- Listening and engaging
- Breaking information or steps down
- Networking
- Researching options
- Explaining or illustrating options, consequences and constraints
- Creating opportunities to experience options and preferences
- Enabling risk.

These strategies reflect the core skills needed for effectively supporting people with intellectual disabilities to participate in support planning, engaging in meaningful activities and social relationships or participating in communities as discussed further elsewhere in this book. Many are illustrated in free online training programmes developed from research at the Living with Disability Research Centre at La Trobe University. See, for example, resources *Develop Skills in Active Support* (Bigby & Humphreys, 2023), *Supporting Inclusion* (Bigby & Wiesel, 2015), *Enabling Risk* (Bigby, Douglas, & Vassallo, 2018), and *Supporting Decision Making* (Bigby et al., 2020).

Training in supported decision making and using a framework such as the one described are important catalysts for reflecting on one's own values and perspectives about the rights of people with disability to make decisions. One mother, for example, said after the training that she would never again see her son as a 'non decision maker' (Bigby et al., 2022). Having a point of reference such as a framework or diagram of the steps also helps to give supporters a structure and remind them to be conscious about decision support.

The Broader Context of Supported Decision Making

The CRPD asserts the rights of people with disabilities to autonomy and self-determination. Too often these concepts and decision making are thought about in terms of the individual and individual ability. However in reality, for people with and without disabilities, decision making is a social process. The CRPD is driving development of supported decision making. It rests on the idea that being autonomous is not the same as being independent and recognises that no one is ever completely independent. Everyone is interdependent on others in their social context. Supported decision making puts into practice rather complex feminist ideas about relational autonomy (Mackenzie & Stoljar, 2000). Very simply, this means that a person's autonomy stems from the relationships they have with others, be they close or distant, enabling or obstructive.

Much of this chapter has concentrated on the strategy of building the capacity of people who are close to people with disabilities and who are often called supporters (paid staff, friends or family members) to offer good decision support. This last section briefly considers other strategies to further supported decision making. First, building decision making skills of people with cognitive disabilities themselves; second, understanding cultural contexts of decision making and third, the role of the more distant others in a person's life—those who work in mainstream services, public or commercial institutions and facilities.

Skills and Expectations About Decision Making

It is clear that good decision support practice also helps to improve the decision making skills of people with cognitive disabilities; as expectations of involvement in decision making rise and participation increases, people will have more opportunities to learn, develop and try out their skills in decision making.

Too often in the past, low expectations of families or educators meant children with intellectual disabilities had few opportunities to make decisions or learn the necessary skills. There are increasing calls to change this and encourage children with intellectual disabilities from an early age to be involved in decision making and explicitly teach these skills. Educators and researchers, particularly in the US, are now developing curricula and strategies for teaching self-determination (Shogren et al., 2015). Learning is a lifelong process, and it is also important to recognise the continuing capacity of many adults with intellectual disabilities to learn not only decision making skills, but also about their rights to make decisions, how to get the type of support they need and how to get the best from supporters. Some innovative supported decision making programmes in Australia are offering decision making training and using strategies such as communities of practice and peer mentoring not only to develop supporters' skills but also those of people with intellectual disabilities (See, for example, Council for Intellectual Disability, My Rights Matter Program, n.d.).

The Importance of Culture

Culture plays an important role in the way individuals and communities approach decision making. For example, in Chinese culture, decision making is seen as the responsibility of the family rather than an individual. For Australian First Nations people, the community is at the heart of decision making which is seen as a collective responsibility. An experienced First Nations service manager explained how decision making occurs in her community, illustrating some of the tensions between western and indigenous cultures:

> We do sit and decide who is going to make the decision and who needs to be involved in that decision-making process. And it doesn't mean that we're taking away the autonomy of the individual. The individual is still centred but the decision is collectively made about what's best for that person. And literally it is our way of doing the circle of support whether you have a disability or not… We hear what they want to – we hear what they say. We know what they mean through either their behaviour, their words and then we'll sit down and have a discussion about what's the best way to support that individual to do what they need to be able to do. (Bigby et al., 2023, p. 418)

There is almost no research about supported decision making in non-Anglo communities or non-western societies. As knowledge develops further, disability support practice will need to adjust to take account of cultural differences in expectations about decision making and good support.

Mainstream Service and Public and Private Institutions

Supported decision making should not just be something that happens as part of the practice of those who work in disability support services. It must also be included as one of the strategies for making society more inclusive of people with disabilities. People with disabilities have contact with many other people beyond their family and disability services, such as lawyers, doctors, nurses, allied health professionals, hospitality workers, train conductors and people who work in banks, or libraries, and so on. Thinking beyond personal to civic decision making, through voting or membership of advisory or co-design groups, people with disabilities are likely to encounter other groups of workers with differing professional backgrounds. In their interactions with any of these workers, people with disabilities are likely to be in situations where they have to make decisions and need support to do so.

Universal design and reasonable adjustments are two key strategies to help ensure that supported decision making is part of wider mainstream systems. Universal design means attempting to make the world accessible and responsive to everyone without having to make changes for individuals. This may be a first step in supporting people with disabilities to make decisions in mainstream contexts. For example, institutions and organisations should

- make information accessible in multiple formats including plain English and easy read—it will help to support decision making about things as diverse as the aims of political parties and health treatments,
- offer variable length appointments to help ensure there is sufficient time for health professionals to explain options and support decision making, and
- build regular breaks into meetings to enable people time to digest and think through their preferences about matters being discussed.

Making reasonable adjustments for individuals is also important. Mainstream workers and professionals can use knowledge from the disability sector to adjust their practice to support the decision making needs of a person with disability. For example:

- awareness about supported decision making, and the need to adjust communication or secure skilled decision support for some people with disabilities, can be included as part of basic training for all public facing workers and professionals,
- modules that teach supported decision making skills can be included as mandatory continuing professional development for professionals, and
- knowledge and competencies about supported decision making can be built into accredited courses and professional standards for key professions (legal, financial, allied health and medical professionals).

Conclusion

Supported decision making is not a stand-alone programme but a set of principles and skills that need to be incorporated in disability and mainstream service systems and institutions. Its progress will be supported by legal and policy reform to set out the legal basis for supported decision making, mandate its use, regulate its practice and safeguard the rights to safety as well as autonomy of people with disabilities. Reforms will shape the context for disability practice, and as the disability sector forges ahead with supported decision making, its work will provide important exemplars of strategies that the mainstream can use to increase accessibility and to make the types of adjustments that will support people with disabilities to participate in decision making.

Take Home Messages

- Making decisions about one's own life is part of exercising choice and control and important to social and psychological wellbeing.
- Rights to decision making are often removed from people with cognitive impairments by laws that determine a person must have the capacity to understand the implications of decisions in order to make them.
- Supported decision making is a new way of thinking that asserts the right of all people with disabilities to make decisions and to have their will and preferences at the centre of all decisions. It acknowledges that taking risks is an important part of decision making which has positive as well as potentially negative effects.
- Supported decision making emphasises the interdependence of all people and the right to support to make decisions. This may range from support to consider options and implications of a decision or support from close supporters to understand and interpret the preferences if a person is unable to express them directly.
- Good support requires time and relies on trusting relationships with supporters.
- The La Trobe Support for Decision Making Framework is evidence informed. When supporters are trained in the steps, principles and strategies of the Framework, they are more likely to provide rights based decision support that reflects the preferences of the person being supported.

References

Australian Law Reform Commission. (2014). Equality, capacity and disability in commonwealth Laws: Final report. Australian Government.

Bigby, C. (2020). Dedifferentiation and people with intellectual disabilities in the Australian National Disability Insurance Scheme: Bringing research, politics and policy together. *Journal of Intellectual and Developmental Disability, 45*(4), 309–319. https://doi.org/10.3109/13668250.2020.1776852

Bigby, C., Carney, T., Then, S.-N., Wiesel, I., Sinclair, C., Douglas, J., & Duffy, J. (2023). Diversity, dignity, equity and best practice: A framework for supported decision-making. Living with Disability Research Centre, La Trobe University: Royal Commission into Violence, Abuse, Neglect and Exploitation of People with Disability. https://disability.royalcommission.gov.au/publications/diversity-dignity-equity-and-best-practice-framework-supported-decision-making

Bigby, C., Douglas, J., & Hamilton, L. (2018). *Overview of literature about enabling risk for people with cognitive disabilities in context of disability support services.*

Bigby, C., Douglas, J., & Smith, E. (2022). *Considering human rights in decision making: Evaluation of the introduction of structured-decision making framework in the public trustee Queensland.* Living with Disability Research Centre, La Trobe University.

Bigby, C., Douglas, J., Smith, E., Carney, T., Then, S.-N., & Wiesel, I. (2022a). "I used to call him a non-decision-maker - I never do that anymore": Parental reflections about training to support decision-making of their adult offspring with intellectual disabilities. *Disability and Rehabilitation, 44*(21), 6356–6364. https://doi.org/10.1080/09638288.2021.1964623

Bigby, C., Douglas, J., Smith, E., Carney, T., Then, S.-N., & Wiesel, I. (2022b). Parental strategies that support adults with intellectual disabilities to explore decision preferences, constraints and consequences. *Journal of Intellectual and Developmental Disability, 47*(2), 165–176. https://doi.org/10.3109/13668250.2021.1954481

Bigby, C., Douglas, J. M., & Vassallo, S. (2018). Enabling risk: Putting positives first. An online learning resource for disability support workers. https://www.enablingriskresource.com.au

Bigby, C., Douglas, J. M., & Vassallo, S. (2020). *Support for decision making - the La Trobe support for decision making practice framework learning resource.* Living with Disability Research Centre, La Trobe University. http://www.supportfordecisionmakingresource.com.au/.

Bigby, C., & Humphreys, L. (2023). Active support training resources. Living with disability research centre and graystanes disability services. www.activesupportresource.net.au.

Bigby, C., Whiteside, M., & Douglas, J. (2015). Supporting people with cognitive disabilities in decision making–processes and dilemmas.

Bigby, C., Whiteside, M., & Douglas, J. (2019). Providing support for decision making to adults with intellectual disability: Perspectives of family members and workers in disability support services. *Journal of Intellectual and Developmental Disability, 44*(4), 396–409. https://doi.org/10.3109/13668250.2017.1378873

Bigby, C., & Wiesel, I. (2015). *Supporting inclusion - online training program.* Living with Disability Research Centre, La Trobe University. https://supportinginclusion.weebly.com/.

Burgen, B. (2016). Reflections on the Victorian Office of the Public Advocate supported decision-making pilot project. *Research and Practice in Intellectual and Developmental Disabilities, 3*(2), 165–181. https://doi.org/10.1080/23297018.2016.1199969

Considine, M. (2022). *The careless state: Reforming Australia's social services.* Melbourne University Press.

Council for Intellectual Disability. (n.d.). My Rights Matter Program. https://cid.org.au/issues/my-rights-matter/

Douglas, J., Bigby, C., & Smith, E. (2020). Building capability to support client decision making.

Guardian and Administration Act 2019. In: Victorian Government.

Mackenzie, C., & Stoljar, N. (2000). *Relational autonomy feminist perspectives on autonomy, agency, and the social self.* Oxford University Press.

National Disability Insurance Scheme Act 2013. In: Australian Government.

Shogren, K. A., Wehmeyer, M. L., Palmer, S. B., Forber-Pratt, A. J., Little, T. J., & Lopez, S. (2015). Causal agency theory: Reconceptualizing a functional model of self-determination. *Education and training in autism and developmental disabilities, 50*(3), 251–263.

Szmukler, G. (2019). “Capacity”, “best interests”, “will and preferences” and the UN convention on the rights of persons with disabilities. *World Psychiatry, 18*(1), 34–41. https://doi.org/10.1002/wps.20584

Then, S.-N., Carney, T., Bigby, C., & Douglas, J. (2018). Supporting decision-making of adults with cognitive disabilities: The role of law reform agencies – Recommendations, rationales and influence. *International Journal of Law and Psychiatry, 61*, 64–75. https://doi.org/10.1016/j.ijlp.2018.09.001

United Nations. (2006). *Convention on the rights of persons with disabilities (CRPD)*. UN General Assembly.

United Nations Committee on the Rights of Persons with Disabilities. (2014). General comment no. 1 article 12: Equal recognition before the law. In *Convention on the rights of persons with disabilities.* UN General Assembly.

CHAPTER 12

'Nothing about us without us'. Including Lived Experiences of People with Intellectual Disabilities in Policy and Service Design

Sian Anderson and Christine Bigby

Introduction

Including expertise from the lived experiences of people with disabilities in the design of policy and service systems, as well as the delivery, review and governance of services, is a growing expectation of communities and regulatory authorities. This chapter reviews the various structures, such as co-designed projects, advisory bodies, board membership and Disabled Person's Organisations (DPOs), that aim to include or amplify the perspectives of people with disabilities about disability policy and services. It considers the types of adjustments needed to facilitate inclusion of people with disabilities and the skills to ensure people's voices are heard when they are present. The chapter concentrates on people with intellectual disabilities for whom the design of inclusive structures and support for meaningful participation are particularly challenging. Too often this group are

S. Anderson • C. Bigby (✉)
Living with Disability Research Centre, La Trobe University, Melbourne, VIC, Australia
e-mail: Sian.Anderson@latrobe.edu.au; C.Bigby@latrobe.edu.au

C. Bigby, A. Hough (eds.), *Disability Practice*,
https://doi.org/10.1007/978-981-99-6143-6_12

either excluded from advisory bodies or when they are present not sufficiently well supported to participate. Although the structures vary, there is much similarity in ways of working that optimise inclusion and support participation. This knowledge is relevant to project workers, service managers and direct support workers who may be expected to set up consultative structures, lead co-designed projects or support individuals who are members of advisory groups or governance boards. For some workers this type of work may be their primary responsibility while for others it is incorporated into aspects into their usual work.

Working Together on Policy and Service System Issues

The United Nations Convention on the Rights of Persons with Disabilities (CRPD) is often seen as the landmark that changed ideas about respecting the voices of people with lived experiences of disability (United Nations, 2006). It certainly drew governments' attention to the value of working together with people with disabilities on broad system issues, that extend beyond their own personal lives. Article 4.3, for example, mandates that all signatory countries should actively consult with and involve people with disabilities and their organisations in the "development of legislation and policies … and in other decision-making processes concerning issues relating to persons with disabilities …" (CRPD, Article 4.3).

However, well before the CRPD, the international disability and self-advocacy movements had organised themselves to influence disability policy and services. In 1981, for example, Reinforce, the first self-advocacy group of people with intellectual disabilities in Australia, formed in Melbourne. It aimed to persuade governments to close institutions, fight for the recognition of the rights of people with disabilities and speak out about injustice. In the absence of more organised consultative structures, Reinforce's initial mode of influence was direct action. As one of the founding members recalled,

> In the early days like in the 1980s well, if you wanted to see a particular person we'd just go up there and sit outside their office, wait for them … did things like occupy the office of the Minister for Community Services [or] squat at a government owned house … to protest the Health Commission's bid to reclaim the house (Henderson & Bigby, 2016, p. 55).

As governments recognised the value of hearing the perspectives of people with disabilities, the focus shifted to finding ways for them to work together rather than confronting each other. Reinforce and other self-advocacy groups became "representative bodies that could, when necessary, liaise and consult with government representatives and other service providers" (Henderson & Bigby, 2016, p 55). For example, one member,

> was the representative on the 1987 steering committee that oversaw consultations about the Ten Year Plan for the Redevelopment of Intellectual Disability Services. Meanwhile, two others attended meetings of another state advisory committees at Government House (Henderson & Bigby, 2016, p 58).

The types of structures established and commitment to involving people with disabilities and their representative organisations in design of policy and services have grown exponentially since Australia signed the CPRD. Their involvement in all aspects of disability policy is now firmly entrenched in Australian federal government policies. For example, Australia's Disability Strategy 2021–2031, which envisions a more inclusive and accessible society, acknowledged the importance of expert knowledge by people with disabilities from their lived experience to achieving the Strategy's inclusion goals. It committed to ensuring that people with disabilities had a 'central and active role' in all aspects of its implementation, monitoring, reporting on outcomes and development of future policy directions (Commonwealth of Australian Department of Social Services, 2021).

The National Disability Insurance Agency (NDIA) similarly aims to put people with disabilities at the centre of all its research activities and evaluations of service design and delivery (NDIA, 2022). This intention is reflected in the National Disablity Insurance Scheme (NDIS) practice standards which expect NDIS-funded organisations to include the input of people with disabilities in governance and have other ways of involving them in the development of organisational policy and processes about service delivery and safeguarding. Since 2021, the NDIA has been leading co-design activities with representatives of its Independent Advisory Council, the Department of Social Services, and 27 disability and carer organisations to identify priorities for operationalising this commitment and ways for people with disabilities and bureaucrats to work together to develop trust and improve scheme processes. One outcome is agreement about the need for a strategic approach to develop and implement meaningful stakeholder involvement across the disability sector.

Co-design is becoming the common term for involving people with disabilities and tapping into their expertise. Very simply, it is a process where the people likely to be affected by a policy or service can contribute their knowledge and perspectives. Co-designed projects require time, thoughtful planning and involvement of people with disabilities in all aspects, that is in defining the problem to be addressed, making decisions about how to develop and deliver solutions, and evaluating outcomes (Reiger, 2020). Effective co-design projects require similar ways of working and support strategies to those necessary for including people with disabilities in structures such as advisory bodies or boards which are discussed in the later part of the chapter.

Why Involving People with Disabilities in Policy and Service Development Matters

Using the expertise of people with disabilities to shape policy and services is important for furthering the human rights of people with disabilities. It is perceived as helping ensure the priorities of people with disabilities drive change, that services are more responsive, benefiting those involved and positively impacting on community attitudes about people with disabilities. From a disability rights perspective it is the right thing to do, although there is only limited evidence about achievement of some of its expected outcomes.

Membership of a self-advocacy group has personal benefits, including learning the skills to speak up, exercising power in democratic group processes, self-confidence, a sense of belonging or purpose, friendships and opportunities for employment (Anderson & Bigby, 2017). Members often have opportunities to participate in consultative and advisory groups, or community education initiatives that influence government policy, and community or professional attitudes. People gain self-esteem and status from these public-facing activities, through, for example, being listened to as an expert by others who are experts in their own fields. This helps to extend their social identities beyond the group to one of 'expert' or 'teacher'. As one participant said,

> I like talking to the people … I do a good job when I tell them the things on paper … I have a practice with [supporter] … then I can tell people all

> about it ... what learning disabled is about. I think those people ... those that hear me talk ... talk about the things, they like it ...it's really quite ... really. Interesting they say. (Anderson & Bigby, 2017, p. 6.)

As well a sense of doing things that matter, these types of experiences also help people to become well known to others in the wider disability sector and increase their social networks. As one member of Reinforce said,

> We achieved so much ... Well, it changed a bit of my life, that's for sure ... fighting for rights more, getting somewhere, letting the people out there know that we're not as dumb, as stupid, as what they think we are, that we've got brains, and we're just as smart as a person next door. (Frawley & Bigby, 2015, p. 259)

The opportunities for multiple social identities that participation in advisory groups and being listened to as an expert offer are rarely accessible to people intellectual disabilities whose diagnosis appears to run deep in terms of social exclusion and negative perceptions. Inclusion has implications that can stretch beyond the personal, in changing not only the way people see themselves but the way they are seen by others.

As the excerpt above indicates, including people with disabilities in shaping policy and services helps to break down stigmatised community perceptions that devalue people with intellectual disabilities, often casting them as vulnerable and dependent. Participation in public-facing advisory groups, events and presentations at high-profile forums such as hearings of the Royal Commission into the Abuse, Neglect, Exploitation and Violence against People with Disabilities or community or professional education sessions highlights people's expertise and challenges negative perceptions. It can mean professionals come into direct contact with people with disabilities on an equal basis as members of a committee rather than the usual unequal relationships, which is also useful for breaking down negative stereotypes.

The value of including people with disabilities as members of boards of governance has been strongly asserted in various Australian public forums including the Disability Royal Commission. There can be little doubt that people with disabilities can enrich board discussions, bringing with them not only a lived experience perspective but also a range of other skills and experiences. Their inclusion can also symbolise the inclusive mission of organisations. Although there is some evidence from other sectors about the benefits of diverse board membership and some research is in progress, there is no evidence beyond anecdotes that substantiates claims that board members with disabilities improve the quality or safety of an organisation's services (Hough, 2022).

Suggested benefits of including people with intellectual disabilities in consultative structures are that their lived experiences act as an 'early warning system' about a range of problems in complex service delivery systems. However, the benefits are often only apparent from the negative impact when groups are left out (Henderson & Bigby, 2018). One example of this is the NDIS. Its design and early implementation included few people with intellectual disabilities and little representation of issues relevant to them by others. As a senior federal bureaucrat pointed out people with intellectual disabilities and those representing their perspectives were largely absent in the consultation and planning processes of the NDIS compared to other groups,

> Probably over-represented and disproportionately represented were people in wheelchairs with physical disabilities who were resourceful, well resourced, articulate, brought to the table a whole set of life experiences, the capabilities and capacities that in fact people with intellectual disability don't bring ... [people with intellectual disabilities] weren't represented in proportionate numbers ... things that were part of original scheme designand quality and practice definitely didn't resonate and weren't sufficiently nuanced ... the original membership of the Independent Advisory Council... There was one woman, a fantastic woman ... she was a mother, a carer,a provider and her son had a significant intellectual disability. But that was a sole voice (Bigby, 2021, p. 262).

As this quote hints the NDIS failed to incorporate issues of particular importance to people with intellectual disabilities—there were no provisions for brokerage or independent advocacy, in-depth person-centred planning or supported decision making or recognition of the long-term or intensive support many people would need to implement plans. This has had significant cost to both the scheme and people with intellectual disabilities and their families.

The design of the NDIS assumed that participants were savvy consumers who could readily communicate their perspectives and preferences. This proved to be problematic for people with intellectual disabilities, particularly those with severe or complex disabilities. The negative outcomes of failing to include this group from the very beginning of the NDIS should inform planning and development of structures for involving people with disabilities in policy or service design, that is that people with intellectual disabilities must be included from the outset. This is a key principle of co-design but too often structures, ways of working and agendas are developed by others without seeking the expertise of people with intellectual disabilities, and consequently the design fails to facilitate this group's inclusion.

Structures for Involvement in Policy and Service Design

Effective structures, adjustments to ways of working and good support are all critical to meaningful and satisfying participation. Various structures are used to involve people with disabilities in policy and service design. Some involve membership of groups, representative bodies, boards or co-design projects while others are part of the work of Disabled Person's Organisations or self-advocacy groups. Some are sponsored by the various levels of government and others by disability service providers or commercial organisations.

Advisory Bodies, Representative Groups and Governing Boards

Traditional structures are advisory or consultative groups or committees established by governments. These include, for example, at the state or national level variously named disability advisory or steering councils or committees, such as the Victorian Disability Advisory Council or the NDIS Independent Advisory Council. All levels of government, types of statutory agencies and private corporations use advisory or consultative structures to engage with people with disabilities. Some structures are focussed exclusively on disability-related issues, such as the inclusion or disability advisory committees of major cities, or transport or police authorities. For example, the City of Sydney's Inclusion Advisory Panel, NSW and Victoria's Accessible Transport Advisory Committees and Victoria Police Disability Portfolio Reference Group. Other structures include disability as part of a broader mandate for consumer or community engagement, such as Local Government Community Engagement Advisory Committees, or Hospital Consumer and Community Advisory

Committees. These types of structures may be ongoing, time-limited or convened for a special purpose. All members may be people with disabilities or members may be a mix of people with disabilities and those with expertise about a particular aspect of policy or other lived experiences. Only one or two members of groups are likely to be people with intellectual disabilities and they are seldom all or a large group of members.

Other types of advisory groups are those that provide advice to boards of service delivery or advocacy organisations. These are known as self-advocacy, client, service user advisory groups or councils and are likely to have a means of directly communicating their views to senior executives or boards. Members are usually all people with disabilities who use a service. They may be supported to participate by staff employed by the organisation or by independent external professionals. For example,

- One of the largest disability support providers in Victoria has its own self-advocacy group which meets regularly to discuss issues of importance and interest to service participants. It provides feedback to the organisation about service quality as well as campaigning about local issues such as accessible public transport. The group reports directly to the board through the chief executive officer.
- A small Sydney-based service which matches people with intellectual disabilities with volunteers who have shared interests, has a user-led group which helps to identify events that might appeal to participants and suggests changes to programme processes. It is facilitated by a volunteer and staff member.
- The board of a national organisation that represents issues for people with intellectual disabilities has an advisory committee made up of representatives from its member organisations in each State and Territory, who provides expert advice on policy and strategy from a lived experience perspective.

In some instances, the way advisory bodies are structured can distance people with disabilities from decision making power, reducing the potential for influence. An example of this is the NDIS Intellectual Disability Reference Group, which has members with intellectual disabilities. The reference group provides advice to the Independent Advisory Council which in turn advises the board of the NDIA.

Boards are governance bodies of not-for-profit, commercial or government agencies that hold decision making powers and influence the strategic direction of organisations. As a group, people with disabilities are very underrepresented on boards, and very few are people with intellectual disabilities. Increasingly, large disability service organisations and national bodies include people with disabilities on their boards. For example, the boards of Yooralla, Life without Barriers, Achieve and the National Disability Insurance Agency all include people with disabilities. Sometimes people with physical or sensory disabilities are joining boards of organisations which predominantly serve people with intellectual disabilities, which raises interesting questions of the transferability of lived experience expertise.

Disabled People's Organisations and Self-advocacy Groups

DPOs are led by people with disabilities, who are also the majority group on decision making structures such as boards or committees. In Australia, some DPOs are funded as peak bodies to represent the interests of coalitions of smaller DPOs. Governments use these types of representative groups as conduits to consult with smaller DPOs or self-advocacy groups about policies, programmes or services. As well as reacting to government requests, peak bodies create their own strategic directions for changes in disability policy or service provision. Some larger DPOs are not peak bodies but represent sub-groups of people with disabilities and undertake activities including individual training, systemic advocacy and representing their membership on advisory bodies.

The NSW Council on Intellectual Disability (CID) is one of the few DPOs that solely represents people with intellectual disabilities. The chair and a majority of board members are people with intellectual disabilities. As a matter of course, CID employs people with intellectual disabilities to work on all its projects, and supporting their participation in advocacy, project and governance activities is 'core business' (Bigby & Henderson, 2018). The organisation campaigns for change on a small number of issues at a time, generating its own initiatives as well as participating in advisory and consultative processes. This targeted approach allows for deep and carefully paced engagement of people with intellectual disabilities which enables their involvement as leaders and spokespeople in the work the organisations work (Simpson & Chan, 2021).

Most self-advocacy groups in Australia are small with membership drawn from their local area and governed by their members. Some are independent and others sponsored by large disability service or advocacy organisations. They are sometimes involved in grassroots advocacy seeking to change local conditions or nominating their members to sit on representative bodies such as local government community engagement committees.

Inclusive Ways of Working and Supporting Effective Participation

These different structures offer opportunities for people with disabilities to contribute to policy and service design, governance or project activities. The success of their inclusion depends on effective processes for supporting participation and contributing their expertise ways of working and practices of support. There is very little evidence about these things in the context of advisory structures or boards, particularly about inclusion of people with intellectual disabilities. However, learnings about inclusive ways of working from inclusive research and support practice in self-advocacy groups provide some useful directions.

The Right Conditions

The histories of self-advocacy organisations provide guidance on involving people with intellectual disabilities in policy and service design. They show that the power to influence policy has been dependant on:

- adequate and certain funding to groups to enable long-term strategic planning about targets for change and offering secure long-term employment for supporters;
- quality of support, to enable participation by members and ensure a sense of ownership and control; and
- a supportive stance by government that means a willingness to listen and act on issues raised.

Yet as the history of Reinforce in Victoria, for example, shows too often funding is time-limited, tied to projects determined by governments or granted at the last minute at the end of financial years. Inadequate and short-term funding results in turnover of supporters and inconsistent quality of support, which varies from exploitative to excellent. Change in priorities or political values mean the governments' stances range from supportive to disinterested. History shows too that even when governments or bureaucrats are enthusiastic about hearing from people with intellectual disabilities, as they were in the 1980s, the inexperience of those involved can mean that at times self-advocates attend advisory group meetings that are inaccessible and so full of jargon and complex language that they understand little of what goes on and barely participate (Henderson & Bigby, 2016).

History makes it clear that if people with intellectual disabilities are to contribute to policy and service design, they require funding to employ qualified staff to assist with determining strategic directions, responding to government agendas and supporting individuals to participate in consultative structures. This fundamental infrastructure continues to be absent from many DPOs and self-advocacy groups in Australia (Bigby, 2020; Henderson & Bigby, 2020). It means that too often the design of advisory structures and support rests with inexperienced staff from government or service providers rather than those with expertise about what is necessary from lived experience.

Building Capacity of Individuals and Organisations

Many people with intellectual disabilities who are involved in advisory bodies or who are leaders in DPOs developed their knowledge about rights and skills in speaking up in public as members of small self-advocacy groups. For example, a cross-national study showed that the self-advocacy groups were often a first step in the process of developing social and political awareness and engagement on the part of adults with intellectual disabilities. Having the opportunity to write one's own identity script (e.g. as a teacher) and embrace the changes associated with this may in fact be an essential step towards confident engagement and participation with the community outside self-advocacy groups (Anderson & Bigby, 2017).

Over the past ten years, since inception of the NDIS, there has been emphasis on building the capacity of people with disabilities to engage in all aspects of community life. This has meant more funding and opportunities to participate in self-advocacy and peer support projects and some targeted projects to increase the pool of people with interest, skills and confidence to join advisory bodies. An example is 'Voice at the Table' led by the Melbourne-based Self-Advocacy Resource Unit. This project aims to increase numbers of people with intellectual disabilities on boards and advisory bodies by building the inclusive capacity of government and community organisation through training to people with disabilities and support workers (Voice at the Table, n.d.). It also publishes 'top ten tips' as a practical guidance to some of the issues to be considered in supporting meaningful participation. Action research by the Sydney-based organisation Side-by-Side Advocacy is exploring the experiences of people with intellectual disabilities on boards and when completed will provide evidence-informed guides to inclusive practices for boards (Curryer, 2023).

Significance of Attitudes and Supporters

The interim findings of the Side-by-Side Advocacy project accord with findings from the very limited research about the inclusion of people with intellectual disabilities on advisory groups that concrete actions are needed to support inclusive ways of working, some people require individual support to participate, everyone is responsible for supporting inclusion and concerns about things such as capacity act as barriers to inclusion (Curryer, 2023; Frawley & Bigby, 2011).

Supporters play important and complex roles in advisory structures and DPOs. Most of the understanding about their roles come from research with self-advocacy groups. This shows that supporters confront difficult challenges posed by power imbalances between them and the people they support. They are continuously juggling to avoid their roles as facilitators spilling over into ones of leadership and control. This requires transparency about decisions and processes and self-reflection about who is setting and driving agendas. As Buchanan and Walmsley (2006) suggest, the inevitability of the power imbalance means sophisticated skills are necessary to achieve participatory outcomes. Supporters must create a supportive space, switching between working in the background creating the right conditions for participation, more directly supporting people, and at times 'writing the script' to enable people with intellectual disabilities to participate in personally powerful ways (Anderson and Bigby, 2020). As the work of CID demonstrates, support to participate must be an integral part of inclusive structures or organisation, rather than added on as an afterthought.

In a study of self-advocacy groups, for example, members and workers saw themselves as working in partnership, having valued and complementary skills. One self-advocate suggested the rationale for the division of tasks was driven by the respective strengths of members and supporters: "We leave it all to the workers here in the office, they know who they've got to ask when we need it ... I've got my other things to do really. I think I'm better for speaking up at meetings and such ... I wouldn't have a clue what to do about the other things [the support worker] does" (Anderson & Bigby, 2020, p. 7).

Inclusive Ways of Working

Knowledge about the adjustments needed to make advisory structures or boards more inclusive for people with intellectual disabilities comes from both research and practice wisdom. There is no formula, as a key feature is adjusting processes to ensure they take account of the needs of every participant. The following aspects of meetings, for example, need attention.

- *Pace*: Pace of meetings or projects should be adjusted to ensure that everyone has the opportunity to follow the discussion or activities and can be engaged in what is happening. For example, care might be taken by the chair to slow the pace of the meeting and the speed people talk or jump from topic to topic. The length of meetings might be reduced to take account of a person's shorter span of attention or the need to rest given the energy needed for some people to concentrate. Short and frequent breaks might be needed to give time for a person to process information or think about or talk through their views on an issue. Hand-held coloured paddles (stop, slow down) are used in some groups so that participants can easily signal the need to change the pace or for a break. A talking stick, that signals who has the floor and should not be interrupted, is another strategy for attending to issues of pace and contributions.
- *Chairing and preparation*: The chair might adjust a meeting's style by including more small group activities that make participation easier for some people or use round robin techniques to ensure everyone can speak. They should tightly enforce protocols about time frames for putting items on meeting agendas or circulating papers so that everyone has time to adequately prepare for each item with a supporter if they need to do so. In project groups, especially if there are long gaps between meetings, members should be reminded about project aims, stages and decisions already made by recapping on progress at the start of meetings and summarising at the end. Careful processes are needed for introducing new members to a group through induction processes and at meetings so that everyone

is familiar with the project or groups' purpose and the roles of others in the room.

- *Accessible papers and communication*: Information about time and place of meetings, procedures, agendas, issues to be discussed and decisions to be made all need to be understandable to everyone participating. Writing in plain English (see, e.g. the Australian Government style manual, n.d.) is a universal approach to making information more accessible. Some people with intellectual disabilities may also need information to be translated into an easy English format. However, individualised support to understand documents may also be required even if these types of adjustments are made. For people with vision impairments, care must be taken in designing and formatting documents to ensure they can be accessible through technologies such as screen readers. If people have communication difficulties, the right technology should be in place to assist others to understand their communication, through captioning or sign interpreters.
- *Milieu*: The behaviour of everyone involved in a project or meeting should support the inclusion of people with intellectual disabilities, both during formal and informal parts of meetings. A key finding about experiences of people with intellectual disabilities on government advisory bodies was the positive impact of collegial relationships and their role in providing a social context conducive to the expression of a range of personal and political beliefs (Frawley & Bigby, 2011).

Individual Support

In addition to adjusting ways of working, some people with intellectual disabilities require individual support to prepare for and participate in meetings. The type and intensity of support always depend on the needs and preferences of the person themselves. In general, it should reflect the following characteristics:

- *Role clarity*: Supporters must be clear about their role before and during meetings. Usually, supporters are not also members of the group and their views about the matters being discussed are not relevant. They should be fully briefed about expectations of their role by their employer, the chairperson, or the project lead, as well as the person they are supporting. It is also important that other meeting participants are clear about supporters' roles as it can be confronting if supporters overstep their role by participating in a meeting or are clearly not providing good support. In either circumstance it is important other participants feel comfortable identifying problems and know who to take them up with.

- *Tailored to the person*: Support must be tailored to each individual and provided in the context of knowing the person and a trusting relationship. Supporters need to know the person they support, their style and personality, for instance, as well as knowing things about them, such as their comprehension, communication preferences, type of technology or other equipment they use and their other support needs. The required values of respect, dignity, choice and control, and person-centredness and strategies to support individual participation are similar to other areas of practice, discussed in this book such as Active Support and Supported Decision Making.
- *Communication and scaffolding information*: Supporting the person to understand the issues being discussed is central to enabling them to consider their own perspective about issues and deciding what they want to contribute. Like writing in plain English or analysing tasks, a supporter needs to break down information into smaller parts and assist the person to go through the information one section at a time. Following the steps of supported decision making, they may assist the person to explore alternative views about an issue or think about the person's own experiences that are relevant to the topic. Supporters should support an individual to understand options and bring together all the information they need to make choices about issues. This process may result in capturing the key things a person wants to say in words and pictures as prompts for them during the meeting. Good chairing of a meeting or project facilitation may reduce the need for individual support during a meeting, although supporters may play a role in prompting a person to speak on a particular item. If unexpected issues are raised by others in a meeting, it may be appropriate for a supporter to quietly talk to a person during a meeting or call for a short break.
- *Reliability and time*: Reliability on the part of supporters is important. Good support relies on relationships and knowing the person, which means supporters are not easily interchangeable. If a supporter doesn't show up, they simply be replaced, but the effects are

detrimental, as they will be unfamiliar with the person or lack knowledge of the context of support. Good support takes time but as it is difficult to estimate how much will be needed, budgets and support workers need to allow for flexibility.

Attending to Practicalities

- The practical aspects of getting to and from meetings, into buildings and rooms, accessing digital platforms and papers, being paid and getting refreshments one can eat are fundamental to good inclusion. Attention to these types of things helps people with disabilities to be confident about their contribution, be seen as equal members of a group, and arrive on time and prepared.
- *Planning*: All the practical aspects of meetings need attention well ahead of time. Planning must take account of each person's individual needs; it means foreshadowing the things that can go wrong and monitoring to check things are going as planned. Clarity about who is leading and coordinating access in general and each person's support is important, as responsibility for different practical aspects may lie with different people across an organisation. The person with a disability must be involved in planning, but negotiation and coordination of these issues should not be left to them unless it is their preference. Importantly, there needs to be one point of contact to call if things do not go according to plan.
- *Getting there*: This requires thinking about the venue and time of day a meeting will be held and the format (face to face, online or hybrid). All these decisions have pros and cons, but the guiding principle should be what will support the maximum inclusion of all participants with disabilities rather than what will best suit the organisation convening the meeting. If the meeting is in person, decisions should be made with each person about the best form of transport to the venue for the time of day. People will need to know about things such as the best entrance to the building, where a driver should drop them off, or which exit to take from the train station. They may need to have been briefed about the location of the meeting room, and any security arrangements such as do they need to check in and get a pass, and how long these procedures are likely to take. For online meetings, testing that the platform and all the technical aspects of connecting, seeing, hearing and talking are important, including

compatibility of computer systems, settings and placement of web cams.

- *Access to meeting papers and other documents*: Documents are increasingly written and stored electronically as printing and posting paper is no longer usual practice. Such changes pose challenges of setting up secure and accessible online places from which papers can be accessed. Assumptions about digital literacy for navigating online repositories, easy recall of passwords and ownership of smart phones for verifying identities need to be identified and managed by meeting organisers with participants.
- *Payment*: Payment for time and expenses are important ways of valuing the contribution of people with disabilities that signals the importance of their expertise. As with access to papers, the manner of payment must be clear and negotiated rather than taken for granted. For example, will the organisation give the person vouchers to avoid the need to pay costs upfront, does the person need to provide receipts and if so, in what format to whom and when, or is there a daily allowance paid automatically? Do they need to claim payment for attendance or are they automatically paid, how do they claim extra time, when will they get paid? If the person receives Centrelink payments do they need support to record and report payments to avoid overpayments? If a person needs individual support to travel, prepare and participate, or for personal care during a meeting, it needs to be clear who is responsible for the costs of this. Should this come from a person's individual support package or is it part of the cost of inclusion that an organisation should bear? These questions are not always clear but need to be asked as part of planning for inclusion.
- *Refreshments*: Sharing food and drink is important in creating a collegial environment. Planning with people about their individual dietary requirements is as important as other practical arrangements. This means identifying needs, ordering food, checking its delivery and ensuring correct labelling when it is served.

Avoiding Tokenism and Other Unresolved Issues to Consider

As already indicated there is little evidence about the participatory experiences of people with disabilities on advisory bodies and governing boards. Nor is there much knowledge about effective structures and ways of working for putting into practice government intentions about the people with disabilities play a central and active role in policy and service design. The little evidence there is, and indicators from other strategies for tapping into the expertise of people with intellectual disabilities such as inclusive research, point to the complexity of the task and failure to realise ambitious intentions.

For example, respondents to a UK survey of participants in advisory groups, research projects and service user groups reported they were extremely keen to be involved but were often poorly supported to do so. In many cases their basic access requirements were either not acknowledged or met. For example, resources such as easy read documents, accessible transport and venues were not consistently available. Unreliable supporters, who did not turn up, only stayed for part of an activity or meeting or failed to work on meeting preparation all contributed to participants' frustrating or unsatisfactory experiences (Batty et al. 2022). Examples from inclusive research projects indicate that people with intellectual disabilities employed as co or peer researchers often feel underprepared and disappointed with both their experience of working on projects and the outcomes of research (Southby et al., 2022). These types of experiences are indicators that inadequate time and resources have been expended in the planning and execution of the project, and that people with disabilities have not been involved in all stages. There is a consistent theme that people with disabilities wanted to have their voices heard and their contributions to make a tangible difference, but when the necessary supports to enable their meaningful participation are not put in place, their personal stories are disregarded and their involvement tokenistic.

Beyond Representation

Questions about representation, who participates and what is expected of them, are unresolved and challenging issues inherent in Australian policies of recognising the expertise of people with lived experiences of disability. While a growing number of people with disabilities are participating in advisory and governance structures, this is still only a relatively small group. A small minority are people with intellectual disabilities, who are usually people with mild rather than severe or profound intellectual disabilities. A central question then is whether people with disabilities are expected to represent and speak primarily from their own lived experiences. If this is the case, then who represents the perspectives of those with more severe disabilities and complex needs than their own? Or are people with disabilities expected to represent the lived experiences of all people with disabilities? If this is the case, then how well are they able to do this? There are no easy answers to these questions, but they are worth considering. They draw attention to the types of voices and perspectives that are not being heard and the other strategies might be necessary to include these in order to complement those of people confident to talk about their own experiences. For governing boards, directors without disability are usually not expected to be representatives, and nor should directors with disabilities. Further, inclusion of board directors with disabilities is not a substitute for other efforts to understand the varied perspectives of people with disabilities.

Blending Different Types of Expertise

One of the core and most exciting purposes of co-design projects, advisory and governance bodies is to bring together people with different knowledge, skills and experiences and distil their individual contributions to solve problem and develop innovative ideas. Tying together different types of expertise and knowledge—the lived experiences of people with disabilities, subject matter experts and evidence from rigorous research that might have attempted to represent the experiences or quality of life of large cohorts of people—is a major challenge. To be done well it requires time and skilled curation and analysis. Such tasks require value judgements about the relative importance of different sources and perspectives, which may not be explicit. While boards are accountable to regulators and constituents, it may not always be clear to whom or how co-design projects and advisory bodies are accountable about the processes of distilling differing knowledge and making recommendations about new policy or service recommendations. Questions about accountability are important and may become increasingly important in the future as more people are involved in participatory structures.

Conclusions

Recognition of the value and importance of including people with disabilities in everything about them represents a major step forward in the recognition of their rights and a shift in the way that the broader community perceives their social identity. Having well-planned, effective support in place to facilitate their engagement in really 'working together' to embed the 'nothing about us without us' imperative into practice is crucial. Including elements such as 'co-design' into projects without fully understanding or being prepared to provide the level of appropriate support to make the experience meaningful and productive for all participants risks inclusive ambitions remaining at the level of rhetoric. It is not adequate to claim a project, advisory body or governance board co-designed or inclusive; it must be planned, designed and executed with people with disabilities. There are added challenges to including people with intellectual disabilities who require more time, different ways of working and more individualised support to participate meaningfully than many other people with disabilities. Providing all these adjustments takes planning, resources and time, but it is vital to realising ambitious policy and improving the quality of policy and services and in turn the quality of life of all people with disabilities.

Take-Home Messages

- Disability policy highlights the importance of working with people with disabilities in policy making, projects and research, and acknowledges their lived experience expertise.
- People with disabilities can derive tremendous personal benefits from participation including self-confidence, feelings of self-worth and purpose, and skills for paid and voluntary work. Their participation can also change community attitudes about people with disabilities.
- Skilled support is essential to ensuring participation is not tokenistic and is a meaningful experience for individuals. Putting the right supports in place, particularly for those with intellectual disabilities and more severe and complex disabilities, requires time, planning, resources and a commitment to supported decision making and engagement in all aspects of the work planned.
- There are numerous organisations which have developed resources to support and train people with and without disabilities to work effectively together and these are a useful starting point for supporters to find out about strategies and tools for providing support which enables people to engage meaningfully.

References

Anderson, S., & Bigby, C. (2017). Self-advocacy as a means to positive identities for people with intellectual disability: 'We just help them, be them really'. *Journal of Applied Research in Intellectual Disabilities, 30*(1), 109–120.

Anderson, S., & Bigby, C. (2020). Writing the script. The overt and hidden contradictions of supporters' work in independent self-advocacy groups. *Journal of Intellectual & Developmental Disability, 45*(1), 1–11.

Australian Government. (n.d.). *Style manual, plain language and word choice*. https://www.stylemanual.gov.au/writing-and-designing-content/clear-language-and-writing-style/plain-language-and-word-choice

Batty, G., Humphrey, G., & Meakin, B. (2022). *Tickboxes and tokenism? Service user involvement report*. Shaping Our Lives.

Bigby, C. (2020). Dedifferentiation and people with intellectual disabilities in the Australian National Disability Insurance Scheme: Bringing research, politics and policy together. *Journal of Intellectual & Developmental Disability, 45*(4), 309–319.

Bigby, C. (2021). "The scheme was designed with a very different idea in mind of who a disabled person is": The National Disability Insurance Scheme and people with intellectual disability. In M. Cowden & C. McCullagh (Eds.), *The National Disability Insurance Scheme: An Australian public policy experiment*. Palgrave Macmillan.

Bigby, C., & Henderson, D., (2018). *Raising the voices of people with intellectual disabilities and changing systems: The contribution of the NSW Council on Intellectual Disability to social change*. Melbourne: Living with Disability Research Centre, La Trobe University. http://hdl.handle.net/1959.9/565594

Buchanan, I., & Walmsley, J. (2006). Self-Advocacy in Historical Perspective. *British Journal of Learning Disabilities, 34*(3), 133–138

Commonwealth of Australia (Department of Social Services). (2021). *Australia's disability strategy 2021–2031*. https://www.ndis.gov.au/understanding/australias-disability-strategy-2021-2031

Curryer, B. (2023). Commentary on governing for quality and safeguarding: What might disability service provider boards learn from others (Hough, 2022). *Research and Practice in Intellectual and Developmental Disabilities, 10*, 42. https://www.tandfonline.com/doi/full/10.1080/23297018.2022.2157321

Frawley, P., & Bigby, C. (2011). Inclusion in political and public life: The experiences of people with intellectual disability on government disability advisory bodies in Australia. *Journal of Intellectual and Developmental Disability, 36*(1), 27–38.

Frawley, P., & Bigby, C. (2015). Reflections on being a first generation self-advocate: Belonging, social connections, and doing things that matter. *Journal of Intellectual and Developmental Disability, 40*(3), 254–264.

Henderson, D., & Bigby, C. (2016). We were more radical back then: Victoria's first self advocacy organisation for people with intellectual disability. *Health and History, 18*(1), 42–66. https://www.jstor.org/action/doBasicSearch?Query=bigby&filter=jid%3A10.2307%2Fj50000335

Hough, A. (2022). Governing for quality and safeguarding: What might disability service provider boards learn from others? *Research and Practice in Intellectual and Developmental Disabilities, 10*, 26. https://doi.org/10.1080/23297018.2022.2109193

National Disability Insurance Scheme. (2022). *NDIA Engagement Framework.* https://www.ndis.gov.au/community/working-towards-co-design

Rieger, J. (2020). *Right to participate: Co-designing disability policies in Australia.* QUT Centre for Justice Briefing Paper, 1–4.

Simpson, J., & Chan, S. H. (2021). From rights to results: Systemic advocacy and leadership by people with intellectual disabilities. *Research and Practice in Intellectual and Developmental Disabilities, 8*(1), 87–98.

Southby, K., Coan, S., Rushworth, S., South, J., Bagnall, A. M., Lam, T., et al. (2022). The contribution of peer research in evaluating complex public health interventions: Examples from two UK community empowerment projects. *BMC Public Health, 22*(1), 1–11.

United Nations. (2006). *Convention on the rights of persons with disabilities.*

Voice at the Table. (n.d.). *Voice at the table.* www.voiceatthetable.com.au

CHAPTER 13

Organisational Culture in Disability Accommodation Services

Lincoln Humphreys

Introduction

Organisational culture is frequently identified as an influence on staff behaviour and service quality. Inquiries and reports into the abuse of people with intellectual disabilities routinely point to the culture in services to explain its occurrence. Often it is argued that by understanding culture then abuse in services can be better prevented and detected. The recommendations in these reports frequently include the type of culture a service ought to have, for example, a "culture of respect" or a "learning culture", but in doing so the concept of culture is reduced to aspirational values and guidance lacking in how to create such a culture. The aim of this chapter is to explain what is culture, how it influences staff behaviour, the characteristics of culture in good and poor quality services, and how to change culture.

L. Humphreys (✉)
Living with Disability Research Centre, La Trobe University, Melbourne, VIC, Australia
e-mail: L.Humphreys@latrobe.edu.au

C. Bigby, A. Hough (eds.), *Disability Practice*,
https://doi.org/10.1007/978-981-99-6143-6_13

What Is Organisational Culture?

There are many definitions of organisational culture, but in essence it refers to shared beliefs, values, basic assumptions, norms and patterns of behaviour that influence how staff think, feel and act. Beliefs are consciously held views about truth and reality. For example, that people with intellectual disabilities can live full lives and be contributing members of society. Values are ideas about what is important, right and desirable, which serve as guiding principles. For instance, that it is right and desirable that people with intellectual disabilities make decisions about what happens in their lives. Basic assumptions are similar to beliefs and values, except they are preconsciously held (i.e., thoughts that are not presently in awareness but can be accessed). For example, staff believe that they share a common humanity with people with intellectual disabilities, but this belief has dropped out of their awareness. For such staff, to regard people with intellectual disabilities as fundamentally different from themselves would be inconceivable. Norms are expectations about how staff ought to behave in certain situations. For example, that staff arrive to work on time and call the service (e.g., group home) or their frontline supervisor if they are running late. Patterns of behaviour are regularly occurring ways of behaving, working and interacting with colleagues and people supported. For example, staff working in a group home eat dinner with the people supported and talk with them about their day.

Key to the definition of culture is that it is shared; there is consensus among staff in terms of the beliefs, values, basic assumptions, norms and patterns of behaviour. Culture can be shared throughout an organisation and among staff groups or teams. When it is shared throughout an organisation, there is consistency across staff. For example, staff in an organisation share the value of supporting people to live according to their preferences. Staff groups or teams can share aspects of culture that are distinct from other groups or teams. For example, senior managers in an organisation agree that research evidence be used to inform decisions about service delivery, which may be different to other staff in the organisation. Or in one accommodation service, staff agree that the completion of housework is a priority and no unfinished housework is to be left for the next shift. But in another service from the same organisation, staff agree that the involvement of the people they support in household tasks is a priority (i.e., Active Support) and not completing all tasks on shift is acceptable. Recognising that culture can be shared throughout an organisation and among staff groups is important for understanding culture and will be returned to later in the chapter.

How Culture Influences Staff Behaviour

Culture serves several functions for staff. It reduces uncertainty and provides guidance in appropriate ways to think, feel and act. For new staff working in a service, culture helps them to manage uncertainties about what to do and how to do it. New staff try to learn and decipher the culture so they can perform according to the accepted ways of doing things and to fit in. For other staff, working according to the patterns of behaviour in the service means they do not constantly have to think about what to do and how to do it; there is predictability. When required, staff draw on internalised values and norms to guide their decisions and behaviour.

Culture enables and constrains staff behaviour by signalling what is acceptable and desirable. For instance, the culture in a good service may enable staff to spend time with the people they support, to get to know them, find out their likes and interests, support them to pursue their interests and identify new opportunities that they may enjoy. That is, these would be considered acceptable ways of interacting with the people they support and appropriate use of staff time. In poor quality services where there has been abuse, physical assault may be enabled because it is accepted by staff as an appropriate response or it is not sanctioned by members of the group. In a study of a service where there had been alleged abuse, new staff were told by more experienced staff to "do the first hit" because the person "would respect you and do as they were told" (Cambridge, 1999, p. 296). Footage from a BBC documentary of abuse at Winterbourne View (Panorama, 2011), an accommodation service in the United Kingdom, shows several instances of a staff member physically abusing a person with other staff present who do not intervene, as well as other instances of multiple staff members working together to physically control or punish a person. In a good service, however, the culture would constrain staff from abusing residents because it would not be considered permissible and there would be sanctions from team members.

Culture is both consciously and preconsciously held by staff. This means that staff can easily identify and articulate some aspects of the culture, but other aspects have dropped out of awareness. Staff may become more aware of the preconscious aspects of culture when they are teaching a new staff member to work in the service, or when they work in another service and have to adapt to different priorities and ways of working.

Characteristics of Culture in Good and Poor Quality Services

Much of the research into culture in disability organisations has occurred in supported accommodation services, such as group homes, and this chapter focuses on those settings. We know from this research about the characteristics of culture in poor quality and abusive services (Bigby et al., 2012; Cambridge, 1999), and some of the characteristics in good quality services (Bigby & Beadle-Brown, 2016; Bigby et al., 2015; Humphreys, Bigby, & Iacono, 2020). Culture has been researched more in abusive and poor quality services, with the intention to prevent and detect abuse, rather than good services, which might inform services and staff about the characteristics of culture they should aim to develop.

Culture in Poor Quality Services

In poor quality services, there can be a group of staff who hold the power and have a strong influence on what happens in the service. These staff may form a core group or faction who support each other and also have influence on new or inexperienced staff. They may use colluding, manipulation or even bullying to influence other staff. A key characteristic of this culture is that the values of the staff group are at odds with the organisation's core values. Instead of valuing, for example, rights and people achieving their goals, staff in poor quality services value order, cleanliness and appearances.

Related to these values are the patterns of behaviour in the home which follow staff agendas. For example, staff cook and clean while the people they support are expected to amuse themselves, which often results in them being disengaged. There is a separation between staff and the people they support. When house tasks are done, then staff may attempt to spend time with the people they support, such as going for a drive to get out of the house and pass the time.

Norms may include the use of excessive physical force to respond to behaviours of concern or simply to move a person. Another norm in the service may be the expectation among staff who work the evening shift that they can finish early when tasks are completed and it is quiet. This expectation encourages staff to finish chores quickly and put people in bed early, and also discourages afternoon and evening activities.

A conscious or preconscious belief of staff working in poor quality services is that people with intellectual disabilities are fundamentally different from themselves and "not like us". They may be viewed as incapable, odd, unusual and even a source of amusement. But not someone that staff would want to get to know and associate with. Staff may talk and interact with the people they support as though they are children, such as singing nursery rhymes with them and using soft toys. When talking about the people they support, staff do so in derogatory ways, focusing on what people cannot do, their impairments or aspects they find amusing. Such staff may mimic the residents or the sounds they make.

Another characteristic of culture commonly found in abusive and poor quality services is that the leadership is poor and ineffectual. The frontline supervisor may have little influence on the core group of staff and be unable to change what happens in the service, or be a member of the core group and part of the problem. Senior managers fail to appropriately manage poor-performing staff or ignore the signs that there are issues in the service. Such services are often isolated within the organisation, resulting in a lack of scrutiny and expertise from people external to the service. Relatedly, staff try to limit visitors to the service, cancel appointments and meetings, and resist suggestions to change and improve the service. Because some staff have been socialised into the service and are isolated, they are unaware of the extent of the problem with the way things are done and how they could be different. More progressive staff who work in such services without sufficient support from their frontline supervisor and managers are likely to leave for another service or organisation that is a better fit.

Culture in Better Services

In good services, there may also be a core group of staff who have influence on what happens in the service. However, a key difference compared to poor services is that staff members' values and priorities are aligned with those of the organisation and disability policy. For example, staff agree that enhancing the quality of life of each person they support is important and desirable. The frontline supervisor leads the staff team and has a positive influence on the culture: by, for example, explaining service aims and priorities, modelling good support, acknowledging when staff work well and providing feedback to improve their practice. The frontline supervisor and staff work as a team to ensure support is delivered according to the preferences of each person supported and there is consistency across staff. When on shift, staff plan together, regularly update each other as the shift progresses, ask each other for help if needed, and notify each other if something needs doing. That is, the culture enables staff to delegate to each other, share information and provide suggestions to improve each other's practice.

In good services, staff believe that the people they support, first and foremost, are people like themselves who have preferences, interests and personalities. This belief manifests in staff behaviour where they spend time with each person, know them, and value the relationships they have with them. Furthermore, interactions are respectful, include moments of fun and a friendly atmosphere. Staff have shared experiences and identify common interests with the people they support, which contributes to the establishment of warm relationships. Staff acknowledge and celebrate when something important happens in the life of a person they support. They feel concerned when a person experiences a setback.

The patterns of behaviour in good services are in essence person centred, which contrasts with the staff-centred patterns of behaviour in poor services. This means when and how things are done is in accordance with each person's preferences. For example, what happens in the afternoon, the activities that people participate in, what they eat for dinner and when, what they do after dinner and the time they retire to bed. In addition, staff frequently provide assistance throughout the day that enables the people they support to participate in meaningful activities and social interactions, rather than waiting until tasks are completed. People are supported to participate and be included in the community—attending places they prefer, seeing or meeting up with familiar people, participating in activities they enjoy—instead of simply being present in the community. Norms include introducing visitors to the people who live in the home and not discussing a person's private information in front of other people. They also include, with consent, sharing information with family members, such as events, appointments and their outcomes, any changes and incidences.

Another characteristic of the culture in good services is that there is collaboration between staff and the organisation's senior managers. This means senior managers understand what it is like to work in the service and know what is happening. They are in regular contact with the service and help staff find solutions to problems. Furthermore, they involve staff in decision-making that affects them. Instead of staff feeling isolated, the service is connected within the organisation and welcomes input from managers, family members and external professionals that will improve service delivery and the lives of the people supported.

Culture and Quality of Life

Identifying the characteristics of culture in good accommodation services is an area of research that is still developing, as is examining the relationship between culture and quality of life outcomes. In the only study that has statistically examined this relationship in group homes, Humphreys, Bigby and Iacono (2020) found that in services where there was more effective team leadership from frontline supervisors, and staff members' shared norms and patterns of behaviour were directed towards supporting the well-being of each person, the people supported had higher levels of engagement in meaningful activities and social interactions. Similarly, they found that when staff norms and patterns of behaviour were directed towards supporting well-being, the people supported had greater community participation.

Their findings suggest that to enhance quality of life outcomes, services should aim for frontline supervisors to be skilled in team leadership. For frontline supervisors, this means that they transmit and embed a positive culture in the service. Some of the ways they can do this have been mentioned previously. In addition, it involves frontline supervisors recognising that they are in a position to shape the service and staff team. Staff are constantly watching, listening and learning from them appropriate ways to think, feel and act. Therefore, frontline supervisors need to model good support and interactions. They need to explain to staff the priorities and expectations in the service, because without doing so, it will be determined by the staff group. They need to regularly teach staff new skills and ways to develop their practice. They also need to use opportunities to help staff to learn from their experiences and their mistakes, by identifying how staff have worked well and providing guidance on how staff can do it better next time. In essence, they need to shape the staff team's beliefs, values, basic assumptions, norms and patterns of behaviour.

Humphreys and colleagues' (2020) findings suggest that staff members' shared ways of working should be directed towards supporting well-being. These ways of working reflect Active Support (see Chap. 7), supporting social participation (see Chap. 4) and self-determination (see Chap. 11). That is, each person is supported to participate in household and leisure activities they enjoy, to participate in their community, to meet people and make friends, and to make decisions about what happens each day and the important things in their life. By working in these ways, people can be supported to experience well-being (i.e., a good quality of life). These ways of working need to be embedded in services as the norms and patterns of behaviour. If they are part of the culture, then it will enable desirable staff behaviours and constrain undesirable behaviours.

Understanding an Organisation's Culture

Before an organisation attempts to change its culture, it is important that its culture is understood. The organisation needs to know:

- What is the existing culture?
- Why the culture needs to change?
- What should the culture be changed to?

One way of learning the culture in an organisation is to spend time in services observing and speaking with staff and the people supported. That is, observing staff work, their interactions with each other and the people they support. As well as observing the people who live in the home: what they are doing, the activities they participate in and their interactions with others. The culture can be ascertained by asking staff about the priorities in the service, what they do on shift and why, about the people they support, how the team functions, the leadership of the frontline supervisor and the support from senior managers. Culture can also be learned by observing what new staff are taught when starting at the service, how staff talk about the people supported and the stories they tell.

This process of observing and speaking with staff and the people supported can be used to gather rich information about the culture in an organisation. The aim is to decipher staff members' shared beliefs, values, basic assumptions, norms and patterns of behaviour. However, this process is intensive and requires time as well as a skilled observer and interviewer knowledgeable on culture. Furthermore, it may not be feasible to learn the culture throughout the whole organisation using this approach if there are numerous services.

Another approach to understanding an organisation's culture is to administer a questionnaire to staff to elicit their perceptions of the culture. There are many generic instruments available which typically assess culture in terms of interactions among staff and work conditions. However, generic instruments by design do not measure aspects of culture specific to disability services, such as the interactions between staff and the people supported.

One instrument developed to measure culture specifically in disability accommodation services is the Group Home Culture Scale (GHCS; Humphreys, Bigby, Iacono, et al., 2020). The GHCS was developed from in-depth qualitative research on culture in group homes which characterised culture in better services as cohesive, respectful, enabling and motivating (Bigby & Beadle-Brown, 2016). The GHCS measures staff members and frontline supervisors' perceptions of culture according to seven dimensions. Five of the dimensions reflect good characteristics of culture:

- *Alignment of Staff with Organisational Values:* staff members' values align with the organisation's core values
- *Effective Team Leadership*: the frontline supervisor transmits and embeds a positive culture
- *Valuing Residents and Relationships*: staff value the residents and the relationships they have with them
- *Supporting Well-Being*: shared ways of working that enhance well-being
- *Collaboration within the Organisation*: support from senior managers

Two dimensions reflect poor characteristics of culture:

- *Factional*: divisions within the staff team
- *Social Distance from Residents*: staff regard the residents as fundamentally different from themselves

The GHCS can be used to understand an organisation's culture, which can inform decisions about where and how to change it. Examining where culture is shared reveals patterns within an organisation. Culture can be shared throughout an organisation and among staff groups.

Integrated and Differentiated Culture

When culture is shared throughout an organisation, there is consistency across staff teams working in group homes. Organisation-wide consistency is referred to as an integrated culture. In a study examining patterns of culture in eight organisations using the GHCS, Humphreys et al. (2022) found evidence of integrated culture in three organisations. In one organisation, for example, there was consistency across their five group homes for the dimension alignment of staff with organisational values. If we were to visit these group homes, we would find that the values of staff in one group home are similar to staff working in another group home.

For staff working across multiple group homes in an organisation with an integrated culture, they would not have to learn and adapt to a completely different culture at each service. Their knowledge of the culture in one group home is transferable to another group home. An integrated culture can develop because of common staff experiences and through aligning staff teams to a common set of beliefs, values, norms and patterns of behaviour.

Identifying where culture is integrated can inform strategies about how to manage culture. For instance, if there is a consistent lack of collaboration within the organisation, then it suggests there is a whole-of-organisation problem, and organisation-wide strategies should be implemented to change the culture.

When culture is shared among staff working in a group home and it is different from other group homes in the organisation, it is referred to as a differentiated culture. In their study, Humphreys et al. (2022) found evidence of differentiated culture in six organisations. In one organisation, for example, there was differentiation across seven group homes for three dimensions of culture. Staff in one group home perceived there were divisions within the team, but in another group home staff did not perceive there were divisions. There was effective team leadership and collaboration with senior managers in one group home, but in another group home, these aspects of culture were lacking.

That culture can be differentiated is probably unsurprising to managers and staff who work across multiple accommodation services. Many managers can identify a service that has a good team where staff work well together, their practices are person centred, and there are very few concerns. But in another service, there are often disagreements among staff, practices are staff centred, and there are many concerns. For staff who work across multiple services (e.g., casual staff), they can work in a proactive and person-centred way in one service, but in another service feel like a domestic worker responding to crises.

Differentiated culture can develop because staff working in one accommodation service interact more with each other than with staff working in other services, staff have shared work experiences, they perform interdependent tasks and have similar personal characteristics (Trice & Beyer, 1993). It can develop because of geographical distances between services, and staff report to and are influenced by different supervisors and managers. Except when an organisation is very small, some differentiation of culture is expected (Trice & Beyer, 1993).

If culture is differentiated in an organisation, then strategies to change and maintain culture can be targeted to specific services. For instance, in the group home where there were perceived problems with staff factions, team leadership and collaboration within the organisation, strategies should be targeted to this service to change and improve these aspects of culture. An organisation-wide approach may be unwarranted in this instance because in another group home these aspects of culture were not perceived as problematic, and therefore there is no need to change them. Rather, in that group home, strategies should be implemented to maintain and enhance these aspects of culture. However, even in these types of situations, organisation-wide strategies should be considered that might prevent the development of significant differentiation between services. These are discussed later in the chapter.

Culture can be simultaneously integrated and differentiated in organisations. Humphreys et al. (2022) found in one organisation, for example, there was consistency across five group homes in terms of staff valuing the residents and their relationships with them, but there were also differences in terms of collaboration within the organisation and the influence of staff factions. Both organisation-wide and targeted interventions are needed in this organisation to change and maintain culture.

Recognising that culture can be shared throughout an organisation (integrated) and among staff teams (differentiated) provides a more complete understanding of culture. Identifying where and how it is integrated and differentiated can inform decisions about whether strategies should be implemented to change or maintain culture, and whether they should be organisation wide or targeted to specific services.

Generating and Reinforcing Positive Culture or Changing Poor Culture

A triggering or critical event can spark a change in culture (Fine, 2012; Trice & Beyer, 1993). For example, a serious incident, a complaint, a change in leadership, the results of a study of the organisation's culture or a significant accomplishment. Such events can provide the catalyst and motivation for culture change to be accepted swiftly. Change processes are often led from the top of an organisation. It needs to be acknowledged that culture change is usually a gradual and long-term project that may involve changing organisational structures and managerial processes, as well as changing behaviours and attitudes of frontline managers and staff, and the "way things are done" in services.

Learning from Cultural Characteristics and Practice

The type of culture in services where abuse occurs is the very opposite of that found in services where people have a good quality of life. Understanding the features of culture associated with abuse is useful in identifying not only what needs to change but also how this might be done. These services are characterised by poor organisational practices, such as a lack of support for staff, negative relationships between staff and senior management, limited staff training, and lack of team meetings or reflective practice (Collins & Murphy, 2022). It is these characteristics that require attention and need to change if culture is to change, and all of these can be influenced by the senior management of an organisation.

Conversely, features of culture in services where there are good quality of life outcomes point to the factors that should be in place to create the conditions for this type of culture. For example, positive cultures are cohesive (effective teamwork), enabling (supporting people to have the life they want), respectful (valuing the people you support and relationships with them) and motivating (staff aligned with organisational values and mission). Although research has not been conducted in how to implement and embed positive culture, strategies for developing good staff practice and embedding it across services learned from research on Active Support and Frontline Practice Leadership (Bigby et al., 2020) provide insight into creating conditions for culture that supports a good quality of life. For example, if staff are trained in Active Support they will prioritise practices that improve meaningful engagement of the people they support, and thus the culture will reflect the dimension of supporting well-being. Similarly, if supervisors are skilled in the five tasks of Frontline Practice Leadership they are more likely to regularly observe staff and give feedback, and chair team meetings that enable staff to share information and work together as a team, which reflect the dimension of effective team leadership.

Influencing culture requires proactive and reactive approaches, which can operate in parallel. First, proactive strategies contribute to creating a positive culture or assisting it to flourish. These are executed by senior managers through, for example, strategic investment in training, new human resources (HR) practices, or redesign of structures for frontline management. They aim to influence who is employed and the way staff in all services work. Second, reactive strategies are used for changing existing poor culture in services. These are executed by senior managers and frontline supervisors through, for example, awareness raising or team development. They aim to directly influence the staff team and their behaviours, beliefs and attitudes.

There is very little research on changing culture in disability organisations, and the following suggestions are based on limited evidence as well as theory and practice wisdom. To change culture, it may be better to identify a few realistic goals that will have an impact. This will help ensure the culture change is followed through and staff maintain focus, rather than trying to do too much all at once. Sharing success stories during the process can help demonstrate the benefits of the change and keep staff motivated. Furthermore, stories are effective for conveying cultural meanings (Trice & Beyer, 1993). Staff working in services frequently share stories about their work experiences; they remember and repeat them.

Organisational Structures and Processes that Influence Culture

A range of proactive strategies are available to senior managers for creating the conditions that generate a positive culture or help it flourish. It is not sufficient to articulate organisational values and mission in clear statements on a website. The values and mission have to be communicated to all staff who need to understand how they apply to them and the people they support.

Value of a Practice Framework

For staff, organisational values must be translated into behavioural expectations that are meaningful to them and their work in a service. One approach is to create a coherent model or framework of practice so there are common ways of working across the organisation. A practice framework sets out not only what is expected of staff and frontline supervisors from the moment they enter the organisation, but also how to do it. It guides staff in a shared direction, with a shared language and skills. Without a practice framework, the right way to work is often informed by organisational policy and procedures, such as medication administration, client confidentiality, work health and safety and so forth. Although important, policies and procedures lack guidance in how to provide support and interact with the people supported, and they are insufficient for achieving goals of enhancing quality of life.

Human Resource Practices: Hiring, Firing and Training

Culture can be influenced by HR management and their proactive and reactive practices. Recruitment is essential to ensuring new staff fit the type of culture an organisation wants to create and maintain. Time invested in this part of the employment cycle to screen people from entering an organisation is preferable to protracted industrial processes of removing unsuitable workers. Interviews are useful for testing verbal competence and whether a person knows about expected values and practice. But they are less effective for judging whether a person can put these into practice. Some organisations use creative methods to overcome these limitations, such as group interviews where applicants are observed and expected to interact with each other and perhaps also some of the people supported in the organisation.

Long probation periods are another strategy for screening out unsuitable staff before they negatively influence culture in a service. Ensuring all staff receive regular supervision can help to identify unsatisfactory staff performance. Performance management can be used to manage staff behaviour that is contrary to the values of the organisation and potentially disruptive to positive culture. The dismissal of staff whose behaviour is unacceptable communicates messages about what the organisation will not tolerate.

Staff inductions should focus on the main knowledge and competencies staff need to know to perform their roles as well as core organisational beliefs, values, norms, and patterns of behaviour. The organisation will need to identify the aspects of culture they want services and staff teams to have, such as those identified as being characteristic of good services. Much of a new staff member's socialisation into an organisation will occur when working in services and learning from other staff. Senior managers can influence this process by determining in which services new staff are first socialised and who they learn from. One approach is to have new staff work in good services and learn from exemplary staff, so they learn desirable ways of working. Once new workers have learnt these ways of working, they can be transferred to another service and receive support from the frontline supervisor and service manager to transition.

Investment in quality and evidence informed training for all staff and frontline supervisors is another strategy that contributes to a consistent organisational approach and shared language. Training introduces new skills or updates existing skills. It should include the practices of supporting well-being, such as Active Support, supporting social participation, and self-determination. Hands-on training for staff led by an experienced trainer and regular coaching from a frontline supervisor can help to embed new knowledge and try out new skills. Frontline supervisors need training in team leadership and Practice Leadership, and senior managers need training in how to effectively collaborate with and support staff teams.

Structures that Support Effective Leadership

There is a growing body of knowledge about the influence of frontline supervisors on service culture and the quality of services. Yet, too often good staff move into these roles without the training they need to be effective leaders. Furthermore, expectations of their role are often too broad, and organisational structures give too little time for the tasks associated with Practice Leadership to be accomplished. For instance, their time is disproportionately allocated to filling vacant shifts, attending meetings and completing administrative tasks. Senior managers must create the structures for effective leadership; they need to give frontline supervisors the time to be present in services to perform the tasks of Practice Leadership and equip them with the skills and support to do these. Some strategies to facilitate this are providing frontline supervisors with training in Practice

Leadership, regular support from their managers, communities of practice, and access to an administration support team.

Service-Level Change

Change at the service level involves the staff team, the frontline supervisor and their immediate manager. For interventions at this level to be successful, staff need to have a shared understanding of the existing culture and the aspects that need to be changed and maintained (Cameron & Quinn, 2011). Frontline supervisors and immediate managers can influence this by explaining the need for change and what it will look like. Rather than challenging staff, it is more effective to bring them along by helping them to understand the reasons for the change and its benefits. For some staff, hearing the proposed changes will be sufficient to influence their beliefs and behaviour. But for others, they will need to "see it to believe it". For example, they will need to be shown Active Support being used to support a person and then try it themselves before changing their beliefs and behaviour.

The process of helping staff understand the need for change can be facilitated through reviewing findings from analysis of service culture, or candid discussion to make visible and bring into the open the usually hidden or preconscious aspects of culture. Gaining an explicit awareness of the culture in their service can help staff to think about what a desired culture might look like, based, for example, on the organisation's core values and mission. It will also assist staff in identifying the positive aspects of culture that need to be maintained and reinforced.

Take Home Messages

- Organisational culture means staff members' shared beliefs, values, basic assumptions, norms and patterns of behaviour that influence how they think, feel and act.
- For staff, culture reduces uncertainty and provides predictability; it enables and constrains their behaviour by signalling acceptable ways of working.
- There are contrasting characteristics of culture in good and poor quality group homes, including: whether the values of staff are aligned or misaligned with the organisation's core values, the frontline supervisor is effective at leading the staff team or not, staff

believe the people they support are like themselves or fundamentally different, staff practices are person or staff centred, norms encourage respectful or disrespectful behaviour, staff are connected with the senior managers and the broader organisation or isolated.

- In disability organisations, there can be similarities in culture across the group homes (integrated culture) it operates and there can be differences (differentiated culture). Integrated and differentiated culture helps to explain why group homes in an organisation can be similar to and different from each other.
- To change an organisation's culture, organisational-level interventions include translating values into practice by developing a coherent practice framework; practices to hire, fire and train staff; and implementing structural changes to enable effective frontline leadership. Service-level interventions include team members developing a shared understanding of the existing culture and how it needs to change.

References

Bigby, C., & Beadle-Brown, J. (2016). Culture in better group homes for people with intellectual disability at severe levels. *Intellectual and Developmental Disabilities, 54*(5), 316–331. https://doi.org/10.1352/1934-9556-54.5.316

Bigby, C., Bould, E., Iacono, I., & Beadle-Brown, J. (2020). Predicting good active support for people with intellectual disabilities in supported accommodation services: Key messages for providers, consumers and regulators. *Journal of Intellectual and Developmental Disability, 45*, 279–289. https://doi.org/10.3109/13668250.2019.1685479

Bigby, C., Knox, M., Beadle-Brown, J., & Clement, T. (2015). 'We just call them people': Positive regard as a dimension of culture in group homes for people with severe intellectual disability. *Journal of Applied Research in Intellectual Disabilities, 28*(4), 283–295. https://doi.org/10.1111/jar.12128

Bigby, C., Knox, M., Beadle-Brown, J., Clement, T., & Mansell, J. (2012). Uncovering dimensions of culture in underperforming group homes for people with severe intellectual disability. *Intellectual and Developmental Disabilities, 50*(6), 452–467.

Cambridge, P. (1999). The first hit: A case study of the physical abuse of people with learning disabilities and challenging behaviours in a residential service. *Disability & Society, 14*(3), 285–308. https://doi.org/10.1080/09687599926154

Cameron, K. S., & Quinn, R. E. (2011). *Diagnosing and changing organizational culture: Based on the competing values framework* (3rd ed.). Jossey-Bass.

Collins, J., & Murphy, G. H. (2022). Detection and prevention of abuse of adults with intellectual and other developmental disabilities in care services: A systematic review. *Journal of Applied Research in Intellectual Disabilities, 35*(2), 338–373. https://doi.org/10.1111/jar.12954

Fine, G. A. (2012). *Tiny publics: A theory of group action and culture*. Russell Sage Foundation.

Humphreys, L., Bigby, C., & Iacono, T. (2020). Dimensions of group home culture as predictors of quality of life outcomes. *Journal of Applied Research in Intellectual Disabilities, 33*(6), 1284–1295. https://doi.org/10.1111/jar.12748

Humphreys, L., Bigby, C., Iacono, T., & Bould, E. (2020). Development and psychometric evaluation of the group home culture scale. *Journal of Applied Research in Intellectual Disabilities, 33*(3), 515–528. https://doi.org/10.1111/jar.12693

Humphreys, L., Bigby, C., Iacono, T., & Bould, E. (2022). Patterns of group home culture in organisations supporting people with intellectual disabilities: A cross-sectional study. *Journal of Intellectual & Developmental Disability, 47*(3), 252–264. https://doi.org/10.3109/13668250.2021.1954482

Panorama. (2011). *Undercover care: the abuse exposed* https://www.documentary-tube.com/videos/undercover-care-the-abuse-exposed

Trice, H. M., & Beyer, J. M. (1993). *The cultures of work organizations*. Prentice Hall.

CHAPTER 14

Building Quality and Safeguarding into Disability Service Provision

Alan Hough and Jade McEwen

How do service providers ensure high-quality and safe support is delivered to every person they support, in every type of service, in every location, by every staff member, and on every occasion? This is the challenge that disability service providers face. If they get it wrong, poor quality support will limit the quality of life of people supported. In exceptional cases, serious harm—including death—can result for the people they support or the workers they employ.

In this chapter, the reader's knowledge is built in stages, starting with a consideration of key terms and core concepts in quality and safeguarding... Stakeholders in quality and safeguarding are then identified and their roles are analysed. The concept of 'levels' for action is then introduced before diving deep into what provider organisations can do to

A. Hough (✉)
Living with Disability Research Centre, La Trobe University, Melbourne, VIC, Australia

Purpose at Work, Franklin, ACT, Australia
e-mail: alan@purposeatwork.com.au

J. McEwen
Australian Institute of Family Studies, Melbourne, VIC, Australia

C. Bigby, A. Hough (eds.), *Disability Practice*,
https://doi.org/10.1007/978-981-99-6143-6_14

ensure good quality service provision. To avoid confusion, it is important to clarify that the word quality can be used as an adjective (e.g., 'high quality and safe supports') or as a noun (e.g., 'the NDIS Commission's role is to promote quality and safeguards'). Safeguard can be used as a noun as in the previous example or as a verb (e.g., 'Building a person's confidence to speak out will help to safeguard them from abuse'). Safeguarding can also be a noun (e.g., 'The NDIS Commission's role includes safeguarding') or a verb (e.g., 'Safeguarding Rahul is a priority').

Understanding the Key Terms

This section introduces four key terms: quality, safeguarding, system, and practice governance. *Quality* is the degree of excellence of something or the extent to which something matches a set of expectations or standards. It involves both the degree to which a person's goals or objectives are met and the way in which they are met. For example, Australia's NDIS Quality and Safeguarding Framework defines service quality as:

> The extent to which a support being delivered by a provider is able to meet or exceed a participant's needs and expectations; and the extent to which that provider is meeting or exceeding the relevant NDIS requirements as implemented under the scheme's quality and safeguarding arrangements ... (Department of Social Services, 2016, p. 101)

Regarding the first part of this definition, some people with disabilities and especially people with intellectual disabilities have become used to poor quality support and thus their expectations may be inappropriately low. Numerous reports by parliamentary committees, commissions of inquiry, and regulators have documented poor quality support resulting in people being harmed in service delivery. Historically, even when the supports delivered were safe, supports were often centred around the convenience of service providers or staff rather than being centred on the individual being supported.

Safeguarding refers to actions taken to keep people safe from harm. The NDIS Quality and Safeguarding Framework defines safeguarding as:

> Actions designed to protect the rights of people to be safe from the risk of harm, abuse and neglect, while maximising the choice and control they have over their lives. (Department of Social Services, 2016, p. 102)

The concept of 'choice and control' used in the Framework denotes that the person being supported has genuine control of their life including choice of what supports are delivered and how they are delivered.

In this chapter, the term *system* is used in three distinct ways. The most relevant use is that of the *quality management system*, that is, the provider's integrated management of strategies for delivering high-quality and safe supports. Another way in which the term is used is to understand *whole-of-system* issues, such as a nation's overall approach to supporting people with disabilities to have a good life. A third use of the term is in *information technology systems* such as specialised applications to assist in quality management.

Finally, *practice governance* should be briefly explained as this term is increasingly used. This term is derived from 'clinical governance' in healthcare, which describes the governance and management of quality in clinical settings. However, for most disability service providers, the term practice governance is more appropriate as the majority of supports provided are non-clinical in nature. The term refers to the governance and management of practice—that is, how supports are being delivered—in disability service provision, with the aim that the supports are high quality and safe.

Core Concepts in Building Quality and Safeguarding

Having clarified the meaning of these key terms, this section outlines six core ways of thinking about and working towards the achievement of high-quality and safe support. These are captured in Table 14.1.

As identified in Chap. 2, a *human rights approach* should inform a provider's objectives and methods of service delivery. For example, Article 19 of the UN Convention on the Rights of Persons with Disabilities declares:

> the equal right of all persons with disabilities to live in the community, with choices equal to others, and [that nations] shall take effective and appropriate measures to facilitate full enjoyment by persons with disabilities of this

Table 14.1 Six core concepts underpinning high-quality and safe support

1. The human rights approach
2. Concern for quality of life
3. Person centredness
4. A commitment to evidence-based support
5. A balanced approach: purpose driven balanced with a management system approach
6. A commitment to continuous improvement

right and their full inclusion and participation in the community. (United Nations, 2006, Article 19)

A human rights approach stands in stark contrast to historical approaches to disability service delivery, sometimes called the 'charity' model, where supports were provided in ways where human rights were optional (Office of the High Commissioner for Human Rights 2010). Under the charity model, people with disabilities often reported that service delivery was controlling rather than offering choices equal to others in the community.

As set out in Fig. 14.1, quality and safeguarding should consider a person's overall *quality of life* (see Chap. 2). Service providers need to ensure that they are providing good quality and safe supports during service delivery while also acting to promote the person's overall quality of life. A person does not have a good quality of life if their needs are met during support delivery but not at other times or if their needs are met in one of the domains of quality of life but not others. In Australia, some of the National Disability Insurance Scheme (NDIS) Practice Standards are framed as whole-of-life outcomes, not just outcomes from the support provided. For example, the NDIS Practice Standard on risk management requires that 'risks to participants ... are identified and managed' (NDIS Quality and Safeguards Commission 2021, p. 7).

Despite the emphasis in Australia's NDIS Practice Standards on whole-of-life outcomes, the NDIS is in many ways designed as a transactional system based on the hours of support provided. However, service

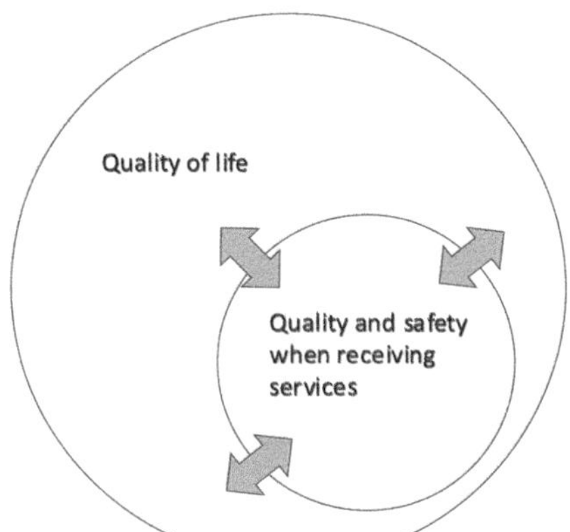

Fig. 14.1 The relationship between quality of life and quality and safeguarding in service delivery

providers should provide support in a way that helps the people they support to achieve quality-of-life outcomes. For example, a person with intellectual disability might ask for help with shopping and accessing community venues. If, in providing this help, the service provider supports the person to build their skills in shopping and assists in building relationships in the community, then the person's quality of life is also likely to improve over time.

The processes supporting quality and safeguarding should be *person centred* and not merely centred around the service provider. Being person centred means focusing on the person being supported, understanding that different individuals will have different needs and preferences, and ensuring that processes start and end with the person being supported rather than with the organisation. A consistent theme in case studies in Australia's Disability Royal Commission has been service providers thinking about quality and risk management in organisation-centric ways and being less focused on the needs of the people being supported (Royal Commission into Violence Abuse Neglect and Exploitation of People with Disability 2022a, 2022b). For example, there were instances of abuse of people with disabilities by staff members where service providers focused on reporting to police and regulators and on the investigation and dismissal of the abusers (such actions were, of course, appropriate) but did not apologise either to the victims or to their families and supporters.

As much as possible, supports delivered should be *evidence-based*. In the last decade there has been substantial progress on building evidence around what constitutes good support in disability service provision. For children with disabilities, there is now a strong evidence base to support family-focused practice, with the professional supporting the entire family in order to provide the best support to the child (McCarthy & Guerin, 2022). For adults with intellectual disability living in a group home setting, research has demonstrated that Active Support (see Chap. 7) is associated with an improved quality of life. For people with psychosocial disabilities, recovery-oriented practice is associated with improved outcomes (Winsper et al., 2020). The other approach which is increasingly adopted, trauma-informed practice, has at this time inconsistent results (Han et al., 2021) and the evidence base is still building.

A provider's quality and safeguarding system should *balance a purpose-driven approach with a management systems approach*. When purpose driven, the organisation seeks to embed core concepts such as human rights and person-centred approaches and to ensure that the design of the quality management system reflects the needs of people supported and staff members, not just those of the organisation. However, management systems typically aim to standardise processes and practices to ensure consistency in the support provided. What is needed is—ironically—the standardisation of individualisation. For example, when planning service delivery, the service provider works with the person supported in a systematic way to understand the person, their needs and preferences, and potential risks to the person (see Chaps. 3 and 10).

One method of systematising the approach to quality is offered by the International Standard ISO 9001 on quality management systems (International Organization for Standardization, 2015). ISO 9001 uses an input, process, and output approach. The inputs to the quality management system under ISO 9001 are customer requirements (i.e., the requirements of the people supported), the needs and expectations of relevant interested parties (the stakeholders; see Table 14.2 introduced shortly), and the organisation's context. The quality management system consists of leadership at the core, and planning, support, operations, and performance evaluation and improvement, using a Plan–Do–Check–Act cycle. The results of the quality management system are quality and safe services and the satisfaction of those supported. This model can be extended to the outcomes that people achieve from the support provided.

However, organisations should not place too much emphasis on management systems for the following reasons:

- An excessive emphasis on standardisation can be contrary to the third key concept of being person centred, as the needs and preferences of individuals will vary,
- What is important is what happens in practice, not the management system itself: the quality management system is the 'means' to the 'end' of good quality and safe supports—it is not an 'end' in its own right, and
- Perceived compliance with standards is only marginally correlated with quality-of-life measures (Beadle-Brown et al., 2008). Paperwork

Table 14.2 Stakeholders in quality and safeguarding

- People being supported
- Family and friends
- Guardians or other substitute decision-makers
- Staff
- Other internal stakeholders such as the human resources team
- Funding bodies
- Regulators

may be compliant, but the people supported may have a poor quality of life.

Finally, an organisation's approach should be based on a commitment to *continuous improvement*. This philosophy recognises that achieving quality and safeguarding is not a 'set and forget' process (Braithwaite et al., 2007). New people being supported, changes in a person's circumstances, new staff members, changes in the external environment, and evidence about new risks to quality and safe service delivery create new challenges. Further, expectations of organisations and staff members will continue to increase over time in response to new and emerging evidence about what works.

Levels for Action in Building Good Quality and Safeguarding

This section introduces the concept of levels of action, providing further insight into how to achieve good quality and safe services. Action can be at the individual level, the organisational level, or the whole-of-system level.

The *individual level* is focused on the interactions between the individual being supported and the individual staff member. For example, does the staff member understand the strengths and needs of the person being supported? Has the staff member been well briefed during a handover or had the time to read the key documents and plans relevant to the person? Has the staff member received adequate training in both generic capabilities and the skills uniquely required to support the person? From the perspective of the person being supported, the moment of service delivery is probably the most important time for quality and safeguarding to be realised. For example, does the support worker respond to and respect the needs of the person at that moment in time, and does the staff member check in with the person and ensure that they are meeting the person's needs and preferences?

The *organisational level* refers to the provider organisation. For example, is the focus of the organisation's leadership on financial performance or on good quality and safe support? Does the organisation's culture genuinely value the 'voice' of people supported (see Chaps. 3 and 13)? Does the organisation follow evidence-based practice, such as Active Support and Frontline Practice Leadership principles (see Chap. 7)? What is the organisation's investment in training and development? Is the quality management system and its associated policies and procedures implemented in practice? Of course, organisations consist of many different hierarchical levels and sub-units and these questions might be answered differently depending on which sub-unit is examined.

The *whole-of-system level* refers to the overall systems of support that impact people with disabilities and their quality of life. These systems include the employment, welfare, health, and education systems. For example, the employment system will influence access to paid employment and thus influence material well-being (see Chaps. 2 and 5). For those unable to find or hold a job, it will be the welfare system that determines their material well-being. To give another example, the wider health system can influence the physical well-being and emotional well-being (in the case of mental health) of the person (see Chap. 8). The design of the overall support system is obviously crucial for people with disabilities. Providers need to have a detailed knowledge of the disability support system and sufficient working knowledge of other relevant support systems.

The Varied Needs of Stakeholders

Having suggested the core concepts and levels for action, this section considers the stakeholders who have an interest in quality and safeguarding. The key stakeholders are listed in Table 14.2.

The discussion below focuses on the individual and organisational levels for stakeholder engagement, although this need applies equally at the whole-of-system level. As will be demonstrated, stakeholder needs usually align, but sometimes clash.

It is fundamental to the human rights–based approach that *the person being supported* helps determine the design of their services, day-to-day service delivery, and the review of services (see Chaps. 3 and 10). Inclusion at the individual level can be premised on the mantra of 'nothing about me without me'. Some providers, especially those involved in supporting people with psychosocial disability, now use the term *person led* rather than person centred to emphasise that they want to ensure the person supported is in charge of all aspects of their support. At the organisational level, the people the organisation supports should be included in the design of organisational policies, procedures, and processes that most impact their interests.

Another important group of stakeholders is the *family and friends of the people supported*, to the extent that the person has social connections with them and is happy for them to be involved. Families and other supporters often have a deeper understanding of the person's needs than do staff members.

Most jurisdictions have a system to appoint a *guardian or other substitute decision-maker* if there is a need for a decision to be made and the person is deemed to lack decision-making capacity. As discussed in Chap. 11, the laws in this respect are slowly changing, but in most English-speaking countries, a guardian or similar substitute decision-maker is required to act in the 'best interests' of the person with disability. The guardian can override the preferences of the person supported if they deem it to be in the person's best interests.

Staff members are also important stakeholders. Frontline staff are tasked with achieving good quality and safe services on a day-to-day basis. Thus, their views should be considered when designing, implementing, and reviewing elements of support to individuals, especially when the person being supported has complex circumstances. The views of staff should also be sought at the organisation level when the quality management system and issues of general practice are being reviewed (Cortis & Van Toorn, 2022). Other important considerations are the appropriate supervision and support, remuneration and employment conditions of staff members, and job quality to enhance the likelihood that staff provide good quality and safe support (Per Capita, 2022).

There will be multiple other *internal stakeholders* at the organisational level. Executive, operational, quality management, human resources, rostering, learning and development, information technology, and even marketing and communications staff (where they exist) can all help promote the achievement of good quality and safeguarding. As discussed in Chap. 7, the extent to which executive management understand and value practice is one predictor of good quality support in group homes. Further, members of the boards of directors and executive teams should provide leadership, including by identifying that service quality and safety are their foremost concerns (Hough, 2022).

Outside the organisation, there will be funding bodies and regulators. *Funding bodies* determine the overall resources available to the person with disability in individualised schemes or, in the case of contracts and block grants, to organisations. These decisions influence the options available to individuals and providers. For example, Australia's National

Disability Insurance Agency makes funding decisions based on detailed assumptions in their costing model about the extent of support and supervision provided to frontline workers and the number of days of training that staff members receive.

Regulators set standards for service provision and can hold staff members and/or providers to account when things go wrong. For example, Australia's NDIS Quality and Safeguards Commission has considerable power, including the right to issue infringement notices, to apply to courts for the imposition of civil penalties, or to ban staff members and providers from providing disability supports. Ideally, the relationship between providers and regulators is based on a mutual concern for good quality and safe service provision, where both parties have a healthy respect for each other and for all stakeholders.

In most instances, the views of stakeholders will align. However, where they don't align regarding individuals, the requirements of the law will ultimately prevail, followed by the preferences of the person supported. For example, a person supported might not want a serious incident reported to a regulator, but this might be legally required.

It is also important to acknowledge that in some instances alignment of views among stakeholders can be problematic. Anecdotally, there are cases where managers of service providers become so focused on the regulatory requirements—whether real or perceived—that they fail to give sufficient attention to the fundamentals of good quality service provision. Another issue is that quality standards typically constitute minimum requirements that must be met, but some providers or staff members consider doing the minimum is enough.

Key Strategies for Providers

Having introduced the concept of three levels of action (the local, organisational, and whole-of-system levels) and the varied needs of stakeholders, two broad strategies for achieving quality and safeguarding, namely proactive and reactive strategies, are outlined. Proactive strategies should be emphasised as they create the conditions for quality and safe support delivery: as the (now very dated) adage states, 'An ounce of prevention is worth a pound of cure'. However, reactive strategies are also needed when things go wrong or 'near misses' occur. When things have gone wrong, the harm caused needs to be corrected. For both near misses and actual harm, it is important to learn from the event and strengthen practice. However, the distinction between proactive and reactive strategies is often a fine one; for example, responding to a complaint is reactive, but providing a complaint mechanism is proactive.

Table 14.3 brings ideas about the different components of a quality management system together and offers some examples.

Going Deeper: What Can Providers Do to Provide Quality and Safe Services?

This section considers in greater detail what providers can do to provide good quality and safe services at both the frontline and organisational levels. Both proactive and reactive strategies are outlined. The examples offered relate to support workers, although the general principles are also applicable to any allied health professionals employed.

Proactive Strategies

Organisational *leadership* is required. Leaders must demonstrate through their words and actions that they prioritise the delivery of good quality and safe supports and that issues such as strategy and financial performance—while very important—are secondary to supporting people to have a good life and to keeping people safe and well (Hough, 2022). Organisational leaders should focus on the overall experience of the people supported and of staff, not merely on compliance with standards (McEwen et al., 2021a, 2021b). Leaders must build an organisational culture that prioritises quality supports and safeguards (see Chap. 13). For example, Active Support is more likely to be achieved where organisational leaders have a shared understanding of the approach and embed enabling factors such as Frontline Practice Leadership (Bigby et al., 2020).

The importance of *observing the core concepts* outlined earlier in this chapter is reemphasised. In particular, executive leaders need to know what constitutes good practice by being informed about the research evidence.

The organisation must build, maintain, and resource the *quality management system*. In the past, quality management systems consisted of policies and procedures and registers, often paper-based. Contemporary understandings of quality management systems are much broader:

Table 14.3 Examples of proactive and reactive strategies for building good quality and safety

	Stakeholder	*Examples of proactive strategies*	*Examples of reactive strategies*
Individual level	People supported	• The staff member collaborates with the person being supported	• The staff member responds to any concerns during service delivery
	Staff members	• The individual staff member is trained in and uses evidence-based practice when supporting people	• After significant incidents, the staff member reflects on what occurred and what they might improve
Organisational level	People supported	• Mechanisms for including the views of the people being supported in the design, delivery, and evaluation of the provider's services are included in the quality management system	• The provider learns from complaints and incidents
	Staff members	• There is organisational leadership for good quality and safeguarding • The organisation determines learning and development requirements • Competency assessments against those requirements are made • Frontline Practice Leadership is adopted as organisational policy	• The organisation responds to whistle-blower disclosures appropriately

(*continued*)

Table 14.3 (continued)

	Stakeholder	*Examples of proactive strategies*	*Examples of reactive strategies*
Whole-of-system level	People supported	• Practice Standards provide minimum standards of support • The system promotes skill development in self-advocacy (e.g., online skill development is available to all people with disabilities) • External quality audit guidelines require auditors to engage with the people supported	• Regulators respond to the complaints of people supported and reportable incidents appropriately
	Staff members	• The regulator provides centralised learning and development resources • The regulator shares knowledge about risks, for example, through Australia's NDIS Commission Practice Alerts • The regulator provides worker screening systems	• Regulator enforcement powers such as the power to fine or ban staff members are used when needed

- Scope: The quality management system must include links to the organisation's learning and development, information technology, and communication functions.
- The customer and staff experience: There is a greater understanding of the importance of the 'customer journey' and the 'employee journey' and of end-to-end mapping of related work processes and workflows. For example, communication with people being supported and staff and access to relevant information are increasingly systematised through information technology.
- Audiences: There is increasing awareness of stakeholder needs. For example, handbooks or guides for people with intellectual disabilities should be prepared in easy English, combining text and pictorials. Policies and procedures directed at staff should be in plain English wherever possible.

- Formats: There is growing recognition that the quality management system consists not just of documents but of visual content such as diagrams and videos. For example, for a person who requires positive behaviour support, there might be a short video recording of a behaviour support practitioner explaining the key strategies to support the individual.
- Automated alerts and controls in information technology: Organisations are increasingly embedding processes and controls in information technology systems, such as automated alerts. These include, for example, alerts when medication must be given or that a person's annual plan is due for renewal. Systems might have 'forcing functions', requiring essential quality and safeguarding data about a person to be entered. Systems can also embed controls, such as an electronic rostering system preventing a staff member without training in PEG (percutaneous endoscopic gastrostomy) feeding from being rostered to provide that support to a person who requires this. At the more sophisticated end, some organisations are starting to experiment with data science techniques such as data mining. For example, data mining might identify correlations between time of day and incidents of particular types, which might suggest preventative strategies.

The importance of understanding *how to foster and maintain good quality and safe practice* is also affirmed. This means that service delivery is being provided by the right person—that is, a person with the right values and the right competencies—who has access to the right information. In addition to the strategies already identified, strategies for entrenching good quality and safeguarding can include rigorous recruitment and selection processes that prioritise the assessment of attitudes and values; frontline and other staff members having a clear sense of job roles and boundaries; relevant learning and development; verification of the competency of staff members; two-way processes of communication with all stakeholders; and sound management systems. Further, good quality and safe practice requires that staff are assisted to reflect on their own practice, receive feedback on their practice, and are appropriately supervised and supported (see Chap. 7). It is also likely to mean that both people being supported and staff feel valued and experience physical and psychological safety.

Organisations need to ***understand and manage risks*** to people supported, staff, and the organisation. These risks include high prevalence risks (risks that are common but often have a low impact, for example, where missed medication is occasionally missed but missing one dose of the particular medication is not vitally important) and low prevalence but high-impact risks (risks that are not common but can have devastating impacts if they are realised, for example, risks of sexual assault). Incidents can have single causes or multiple contributing factors. Further, risk management needs to embrace the idea of building in multiple protections rather than a single protection such as relying on a staff member's memory or supposed competence. However, for every protection put in place, there will also be 'holes' in those protections; unexpected incidents happen when the holes in those protections align; this is the basis of James Reason's 'Swiss Cheese' model of incident causation and prevention (Reason, 1997).

Risks to people supported can be classified as risks of abuse (Collins & Murphy, 2022) or risks of neglect. The risks can be at the personal level, or they can be systemic, that is built into the service system at a local or whole-of-system level. An example of abuse at the person level would be violence by a staff member towards a person supported. An example of organisationally systemic abuse could be a service provider having low expectations about what the people they support can achieve and acting on those low expectations. An example of individual neglect would be failing to support a person with a profound intellectual disability to engage in or to attend to their hydration needs. Organisational systemic neglect would be designing the service system around the needs of the organisation and not the needs of the people supported.

Risks to staff will range from the classic 'slips, trips, and falls' to motor vehicle incidents. In addition, without wishing to overstate these risks, there can be risks associated with the challenging behaviours of people supported.

Risks to people supported and to staff create *risks to the organisation*. These include compliance risks (e.g., not complying with legal obligations) and reputational risks. Organisations can themselves create risks, such as when the organisation is growing too quickly, providing new types of supports, or providing support in new locations without remediation of the risks associated with changes to services.

The examples offered above have focused on the negative aspects of risk. However, some risks can be positive, such as when a person being supported is developing new skills or new relationships. Thus, there is a role for what is known as risk enablement. Consistent with the concept of dignity of risk, people have the right to take risks in their lives, provided that the individual team member and the providers' duties of care are not breached. In most instances, both dignity of risk and duty of care can be achieved.

There need to be proactive strategies to ***understand how well support is being delivered***. At the individual level, this may include checking with the individual supported about the quality and safety of the supports provided if they are able to provide feedback, or else observing the support or seeking perspectives of families and supporters. At the organisational level, strategies include internal reporting, standard performance measures such as the experience of those using services and their personal outcomes, staff experience, and matters such as the completion of essential training. Observation of actual practice is one of the elements of Frontline Practice Leadership (see Chap. 7) with feedback provided to staff members about their practice. Internal and external quality audits can be other valuable sources of information, although these will be more useful if they focus on actual practice and not merely on paper-based compliance (McEwen et al., 2014, 2020). Further, external quality audits can sometimes fail to identify abusive cultures (Murphy, 2020). External and regular evaluation of the quality and safety of supports being provided can be another useful strategy. Some countries have 'official visitor' schemes where an external visitor is appointed by the government to visit settings such as group homes. Some providers have established the internal equivalent of official visitors, including the use of peer quality checkers.

Reactive Strategies

There are two main sources of reactive strategies: first, complaints and other feedback and, second, incidents. *Complaints* provide information on where the service provider is perceived not to have performed well. Of course, *feedback* can also be positive, providing information on where the staff member or the organisation is perceived to have done well. While staff and organisations sometimes respond defensively to negative feedback, it is better to start with the assumption that such feedback is an opportunity to learn and improve. Likewise, whistle-blower disclosure mechanisms can give the provider information that it might not otherwise receive through usual lines of reporting.

The second use of reactive strategies is in response to ***incidents***, including incidents that must be reported to regulators. Incident reporting discloses significant events that have occurred for people supported, staff, or any other people involved which can relate to the quality and safety of the support being provided.

For both complaints and incidents, the first response is to check that people are safe and, if not, to ensure their safety. If police or regulators must be notified immediately, this is the organisation's next step. Next, the provider needs to establish the facts of what occurred, which might be done in lesser or greater detail depending on the seriousness of the incident. Sometimes it is enough to establish merely the core facts, but at other times a formal investigation might be commissioned, for example, if an allegation is made that a person using services has been assaulted.

Other reactive strategies vary and may overlap with one another. Australia's NDIS Quality and Safeguards Commission recommends practice review as one response. Some commentators believe in the importance of 'root cause' analysis, using methods such as the 'five whys': asking 'why' something happened five times in succession to establish the root cause. This is illustrated in Table 14.4.

Some commentators believe that processes such as learning teams, bringing frontline staff members and technical experts together to learn from experience, are more useful (Dekker & Conklin, 2022). One option for learning teams is to review what caused good practice, not merely what has resulted in poor practice.

Consistent with the philosophy of being person centred, one of the requirements of Australia's NDIS Quality and Safeguards Commission for both complaints and incidents is that the people with disabilities involved or affected must be involved in the resolution of the issues. Further, the Commission requires periodic reviews of issues arising and reviews of the

Table 14.4 An example of applying the five 'whys'

Example: Maggie, who uses a wheelchair and cannot use her arms to control the wheelchair was injured because the wheelchair brakes were not applied effectively by her support worker, Fran. Maggie rolled down an incline and was injured.
Why? The brakes were not applied effectively.
Why? The brake pads had become worn.
Why? Maggie had not ensured that the wheelchair was properly maintained (in this case assuming that she was responsible for maintenance).
Why? Maggie needs support and funding for regular wheelchair maintenance.
Why? No one has explained to Maggie the need for wheelchair maintenance.

effectiveness of the management systems supporting complaints and incidents.

When things do go wrong, one of the dilemmas that providers must confront is the degree to which their focus is on the attribution of blame or on learning. This is not necessarily an easy dilemma to resolve. On the one hand, if a person who receives services is harmed by the deliberate actions or neglect of a staff member, then the person harmed and the community rightly expect that the staff member will be held accountable. On the other hand, if staff are blamed—or perceive that they will be blamed—for errors that arise from the system of work or at the organisational level (e.g., inadequate training), or because of judgments that had to be made on the run in difficult circumstances, this will have the unintended consequence of reducing the staff members' willingness to report incidents and near misses. This will ultimately reduce the capacity to learn from events (Reason, 2000).

Conclusion

Let us end where we started. Every year, people with disabilities and staff members are seriously harmed and even die because of poor quality or unsafe service delivery. This harm is often preventable. The challenge that service providers face is that they must attempt to ensure that every occasion of service delivery is of good quality and is safe, despite working in dynamic environments where the needs of people can quickly change. As the saying goes, 'Wisdom in hindsight is the least useful form of wisdom'. The puzzle that service providers and managers must attempt to solve is how to build 'wisdom in anticipation'. The authors' hope is that this chapter and the other chapters of this book have contributed ideas towards such wisdom in advance.

Take Home Messages

- Six core concepts should underpin good quality and safeguarding: the human rights approach; a focus on quality of life; person centredness; a commitment to evidence-based practice; a balance between purpose-driven and management system approaches; and dedication to continuous improvement.
- In many areas of disability support provision, we now have research evidence about what constitutes good practice.

- Building good quality and safeguarding into disability service provision requires both proactive and reactive approaches at the individual, organisational, and service system levels.
- Stakeholders' needs about quality and safeguarding usually align; however, sometimes they vary. Where they vary, the ultimate determining factor is what is legally required of the provider and staff member.
- Many different strategies are needed to achieve good quality and safeguarding, including leadership, and building an appropriate organisational culture.
- The common approach to managing quality in organisations is to build and implement a quality management system. Quality management systems should have processes that are user-friendly for the people being supported, their families and supporters, staff members, and organisations.
- Quality management systems can contribute to good quality and safeguarding but are not adequate to assure these in and of themselves.

Acknowledgement The authors gratefully acknowledge Servena McIntyre for her advice about the proposed content of this chapter and Jenny Klause for her comments on the draft. Responsibility for the chapter's content rests with the authors.

References

Beadle-Brown, J., Hutchinson, A., & Mansell, J. (2008). Care standards in homes for people with intellectual disabilities. *Journal of Applied Research in Intellectual Disabilities, 21*(3), 210–218. https://doi.org/10.1111/j.1468-3148.2007.00400.x

Bigby, C., Bould, E., Iacono, T., & Beadle-Brown, J. (2020). Quality of practice in supported accommodation services for people with intellectual disabilities: What matters at the organisational level. *Journal of Intellectual and Developmental Disability, 45*(3), 290–302. https://doi.org/10.3109/13668250.2019.1671965

Braithwaite, J., Makkai, T., & Braithwaite, V. (2007). *Regulating aged care: Ritualism and the new pyramid*. Edward Elgar.

Collins, J., & Murphy, G. H. (2022). Detection and prevention of abuse of adults with intellectual and other developmental disabilities in care services: A systematic review. *Journal of Applied Research in Intellectual Disabilities, 35*(2), 338–373. https://doi.org/10.1111/jar.12954

Cortis, N., & Van Toorn, G. (2022). Safeguarding in Australia's new disability markets: Frontline workers' perspectives. *Critical Social Policy, 42*, 197–219. https://doi.org/10.1177/02610183211020693

Dekker, S., & Conklin, T. (2022). *Do safety differently*. Pre Accident Media.

Department of Social Services. (2016). *NDIS quality and safeguarding framework*. Australian Government.

Han, H., Miller, H. N., Nkimbeng, M., Budhathoki, C., Mikhael, T., Rivers, E., Gray, J. L., Trimble, K., Chow, S., & Wilson, P. (2021). Trauma informed interventions: A systematic review. *PLoS One, 16*(6), e0252747. https://doi.org/10.1371/journal.pone.0252747

Hough, A. (2022). Governing for quality and safeguarding: What might disability service provider boards learn from others? *Research and Practice in Intellectual and Developmental Disabilities*. https://doi.org/10.1080/23297018.2022.2109193

International Organization for Standardization. (2015). ISO9001: Quality management systems: Requirements. ISO.

McCarthy, E., & Guerin, S. (2022). Family-centred care in early intervention: A systematic review of the processes and outcomes of family-centred care and impacting factors. *Child: Care, Health and Development, 48*(1), 1–32. https://doi.org/10.1111/cch.12901

McEwen, J., Bigby, C., & Douglas, J. (2014). What are Victoria's disability service standards really measuring? *Research and Practice in Intellectual and Developmental Disabilities, 1*(2), 148–159. https://doi.org/10.1080/23297018.2014.956385

McEwen, J., Bigby, C., & Douglas, J. (2020). Moving on from quality assurance: Exploring systems that measure both process and personal outcomes in disability services. *Journal of Policy and Practice in Intellectual Disabilities, 17*(4), 364–375. https://doi.org/10.1111/jppi.12295

McEwen, J., Bigby, C., & Douglas, J. (2021a). How leaders in day service organisations understand service quality. *Research and Practice in Intellectual and Developmental Disabilities, 8*(2), 126–134. https://doi.org/10.1080/23297018.2021.1951619

McEwen, J., Bigby, C., & Douglas, J. (2021b). What is good service quality? Day service staff's perspectives about what it looks like and how it should be monitored. *Journal of Applied Research in Intellectual Disabilities, 34*(4), 1118–1126. https://doi.org/10.1111/jar.12871

Murphy, G. (2020). *CQC inspections and regulation of Whorlton Hall: Second independent report*. Care Quality Commission.

NDIS Quality and Safeguards Commission (2021). NDIS Practice Standards and Quality Indicators, *Version 4*.

Office of the High Commissioner for Human Rights (2010). Monitoring the convention on the rights of persons with disabilities: Guidance for human rights monitors. United Nations.

Per Capita. (2022). *Contracting care: The rise and risks of digital contractor work in the NDIS* [Report]. https://apo.org.au/node/318417.

Reason, J. (1997). *Managing the risks of organizational accidents*. Routledge.

Reason, J. (2000). Safety paradoxes and safety culture. *Injury Control & Safety Promotion, 7*(1), 3–14.

Royal Commission into Violence Abuse Neglect and Exploitation of People with Disability (2022a). *Public Hearing Report: Public hearing 13 - Preventing and responding to violence, abuse, neglect and exploitation in disability services (a Case Study)*.

Royal Commission into Violence Abuse Neglect and Exploitation of People with Disability (2022b). *Public Hearing Report: Public hearing 14 - Preventing and responding to violence, abuse, neglect and exploitation in disability services (South Australia)*.

United Nations. (2006). *Convention on the rights of persons with disabilities (CRPD)*. UN General Assembly.

Winsper, C., Crawford-Docherty, A., Weich, S., Fenton, S. J., & Singh, S. P. (2020). How do recovery-oriented interventions contribute to personal mental health recovery? A systematic review and logic model. *Clinical Psychology Review, 76*, 101815. https://doi.org/10.1016/j.cpr.2020.101815

Index

A

C. Bigby, A. Hough (eds.), *Disability Practice*,
https://doi.org/10.1007/978-981-99-6143-6

SPRINGER NATURE

GPSR Compliance

The European Union's (EU) General Product Safety Regulation (GPSR) is a set of rules that requires consumer products to be safe and our obligations to ensure this.

If you have any concerns about our products, you can contact us on ProductSafety@springernature.com

In case Publisher is established outside the EU, the EU authorized representative is:

Springer Nature Customer Service Center GmbH
Europaplatz 3
69115 Heidelberg, Germany

The manufacturer's authorised representative in the EU is Springer Nature Customer Service Centre GmbH, Europaplatz 3, 69115 Heidelberg, Germany. If you have any concerns regarding our products, please contact ProductSafety@springernature.com

Printed and bound by CPI Group (UK) Ltd, Croydon, CR0 4YY
30/09/2026
02225321-0009